THE SIMPLE PLAN

THE SIMPLE PLAN

7 HABITS FOR HEALTHY LIVING

DR. CHRIS PERRON

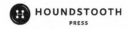

HOUNDSTOOTH
PRESS

COPYRIGHT © 2022 CHRIS PERRON

THE SIMPLE PLAN

7 Habits for Healthy Living

FIRST EDITION

ISBN   978-1-5445-3529-6 *Hardcover*

978-1-5445-3530-2 *Paperback*

978-1-5445-3531-9 *Ebook*

To my family, my "primary" patients, whom I love.

My mother, Claudia, for whom this plan was literally created to help.

My father, Richard, because I would like to keep him around as long as possible, too.

My children, Becca and Matthew, for their unconditional love and support. You both are the greatest gifts in my life.

CONTENTS

INTRODUCTION

On Monday, June 8, 2020, I finished taking care of patients for the morning and went into my private office. I grabbed my phone and keys to go home for lunch. I looked at my phone, and it read "Missed Call Dad Perron." I thought, *That's odd*. It was the first time I could recall my father calling my cell phone. My parents usually call my house after office hours, when they know I am available.

I decided to call him back from my truck on my four-mile drive home. But before I made it to my truck I got a text from my younger sister, Catherine. "Have you talked to Dad yet? You need to call him right away!"

Immediately my heart jumped, and a lump appeared in my throat. Now I was worried. Not really wanting to call, for fear of what I was about to hear, I pressed "Call Back."

My dad answered. He was sitting in a hospital parking lot, choking back tears. His lips trembled as he filled me in. "Your mother just had a heart attack. They called this kind of heart attack 'The Widowmaker.' They told me that she is stable now and we are lucky we got here when we did, but I can't even go in to see her because of COVID-19 restrictions."

Thank God everything had come together perfectly. He relayed that my mom did not feel "right" that morning and told him to call 911. He suggested that she take a moment, but she insisted and he obliged. By the time the emergency medical technicians (EMTs) arrived at my parents' house, a few minutes later, things had begun to get worse. They put her on a board, strapped her down and wheeled her out the front door of the house, and loaded her in the back of the ambulance. As they sped to the hospital with lights flashing and sirens wailing, they evaluated and treated her to the extent they could. The EMTs sent their test results to the hospital electronically en route, so when the ambulance arrived, the hospital staff wheeled my mom straight to the operating room where the doctors performed emergency procedures.

My mom was only sixty-nine!

She was not on any medications; although she, like most people, could stand to lose a few pounds and be more active.

Nonetheless, she was considered to be a "fairly healthy" person by her doctors.

Just two days before, on June 6, my two sisters and our families logged on to a Zoom meeting to celebrate my parents' 50th wedding anniversary. Although it was a major step down from the family reunion we had planned on Hilton Head Island, it was still good to get everyone together. *Was that going to be the last time I saw my mom?*

She was fortunate! Everything came together and she survived. This of course was great news, but it did not negate the fact that she *almost died* of a heart attack!

This was a *big* eye opener for her and my father. You see, we don't really know what challenges our health might bring us. Health issues can seem sudden, though I have found that it is typically the culmination of factors over several years finally reaching a tipping point and bringing them to the surface.

With the COVID-19 pandemic in full swing, my mother was not allowed to have any visitors in the hospital. I had to wait to see her. She was released from the hospital two days later (on a Wednesday), but it felt like two weeks.

FINDING A BETTER WAY

I drove down to South Carolina from my home in the suburbs of Washington, DC, the day after her release.

As a healthcare professional myself—a Doctor of Chiropractic—I wanted to see what I could provide to help my mom. I also wanted to offer my parents a plan to help them know how to improve their general health and decrease their chances of going through this again.

I drove my gold Ford F-150 south on Interstate 95 for nine hours, by myself. The whole time I was racking my brain, thinking, *How can I share what is in my head with my parents? It makes sense to me after twenty-four years of caring for thousands of patients and seeing what works and what doesn't work. But how can I put all that information into a simple plan that they can understand and use, without me having to be there? A plan that is practical so that it can realistically be followed for the long term, not just a temporary bandage.*

One thing has been a consistent truth in my now twenty-six years of caring for patients: *real health is about the long game.* We can all do good things for a stretch of time and that is good. And we can all fall off the good path for a stretch of time, and in most cases, that is not the end of the world either. But it is really the overall trend of how we live, and the choices we make, that has the greatest impact on our health. As I drove, I organized my ideas into seven simple habits.

I pulled into my parents' driveway at the end of the cul de sac in the Sun City retirement community where they had lived for the past ten years. My dad greeted me at the door. There were hugs and mostly a feeling of relief. I examined my mother and gave her a chiropractic adjustment to reduce the strain that her heart attack had clearly put on her body. Then, after catching up on the details of the saga, I sat down at the kitchen counter and wrote out my plan. It only took about thirty minutes to get the framework out and establish the primary points. Next, I needed to get their buy-in.

THE SIMPLE PLAN

There is another truth that I have come to recognize over the course of my career: *nobody can really help you; you must want to help yourself.* Even if I am the doctor performing the treatment, the patient still must show up when advised and put forth some effort at home to support the process of building their health.

I wanted to help my parents, but they would have to want to help themselves, too. "Mom and Dad, if you are open to it, I have some suggestions I would like to share with you to help you be healthier. Would you be interested in my help?" I was relieved that they were extremely open, and motivated to take on this plan. Right at that moment, they became my test subjects for what would come to be called The Simple Plan.

This book contains the same seven habits I outlined for them. This information was never intended to become anything other than trying to help my mom live longer. You'll be reading the exact advice I gave my own Mom and Dad. Wait until you see the results!

Have you experienced a health scare like my mom? Have you had a loved one experience something similar? Even if you just want to avoid your own health scare, then keep reading.

Over the course of the next three days, we talked about the plan, and I made sure that they understood it. I took my dad grocery shopping, which was clearly a foreign activity to him, but in no time he became a pro. I tweaked things that weren't clear to them. Then, off I went to return to my home, leaving behind the best I had to offer in the form of 7 Habits for Healthy Living.

Fast forward four months, they had dropped a combined total of seventy-six pounds! They went to their doctors, my mother for a follow-up after her heart attack and my father for his general annual checkup. Their doctors barely recognized them as their blood work had changed so much and the way they looked was so different.

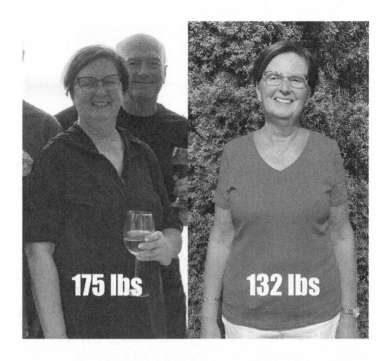

My parents can tell you how much better they feel, and it was all from following the 7 Habits for Healthy Living. The seven habits are intended to be a package deal. However, the first two (Incorporating Chiropractic Care and Restoring Your Gut and Brain) are both targeted at fixing damage already done and getting back to as close of a clean slate as possible. I'm Catholic, so I refer to it as "forgiving you for your past sins." From there, you can move forward with a clean (or at least much cleaner) slate. The other five habits are about day-to-day living and being healthy overall for the long term. To help you remember the habits, I made the acronym FRESH. The FRESH five are:

Food (Feed Your Body)

Rest (Prioritize Rest and Recovery)

Exercise (Be Active!)

Self-Love (Cultivate the Mindset to Succeed)

Hydration (Drink Up!)

The habits are simple to follow and purposely not complex. *The subjects* are complex, *your body* is complex, but the plan is not, and that is the point of me sharing this with you. Complexity is a deterrent to action, but a plan that is simple to follow gives you a real opportunity for success.

TWO PHASES OF THE SIMPLE PLAN

PHASE ONE: 90 DAY TRANSFORMATION PROGRAM

This program is an intensive of what is outlined in *The Simple Plan*. I strongly advise you to start with this program to really reset your entire system and allow you to adopt these new healthy habits and replace old habits that were not serving you well.

Science has shown that it takes three weeks to incorporate a habit, consciously. Which means you still have to think about it to keep it going and that means effort and focus.

It takes sixty days to make this habit sink into your subconscious. Which means it still takes *some* effort but less effort to keep things going. However, at ninety days you have created an automatic feedback loop in your neurology where you are on autopilot. You still have choices to make each day, as always, but you are so in the groove at this point that there is minimal effort to keep going. In fact, it can take more effort to go back to old habits. This is your goal and that is why you need to sustain for ninety days to achieve this level of habit.

The 90 Day Transformation Program incorporates all seven habits simultaneously, which is ideal, and is also how you get extremely good results. This timeline will include the 90 Day Gut and Brain Restoration Program and eating exceptionally well. Eating plenty, but eating quality, healthy food. It is everything that I will outline in this book (but no cheating!), for at least ninety days.

This will be challenging. Not because it is confusing—it is The Simple Plan—but because it requires change. Change is hard for everyone. To support your effort, I created The Simple Plan community, as part of my private coaching programs. The Simple Plan Community is anchored by my weekly webinar, *Dr. Perron's Office Hours*. This is a consistent time and place to log in from anywhere in the world and have your questions answered and gain a better understanding of why and how this all works. Most of all, you get to see that you are not alone on this journey and exchange encouragement and empathy with others just like you. I offer coaching programs to assist you further in this transition for the fastest and best results. Life is short; the fastest path to your best quality of life is what I am on a mission to deliver. The concepts in this book are already proven to work, but it is the implementation into your life that will give them value. This book is meant to give you all the information, but many people have requested additional guidance in their real world to expedite their results, so I created the coaching programs to meet this desire.

You can find more on these options at www.ChrisPerron. com.

PHASE TWO: THE SIMPLE PLAN LIFESTYLE

This phase begins once you have achieved your cruising speed. Where you want to be with regard to your health and then staying there is actually the easier part. If you followed the instructions in entirety for at least ninety days, then you will have reset your brain. You want to continue with your new habits, but skip the stress or guilt when you are traveling or just out to dinner with friends. My parents went out to a coffee shop they loved to go to pre–heart attack to celebrate my father's birthday, which happened to be a few days after their ninety days ended. They ordered this enormous, freshly baked blueberry muffin they loved. I said,

"Seriously?! That is about the worst thing to start with, but how did it go?" My mom said, "You know, it was not as good as I remembered." Sweet! Their taste buds had changed. Since then they have gone to Hawaii for weeks at a time and other travel and by default eaten out a lot during those times and guess what? They have maintained their results.

The Simple Plan Lifestyle does not include stress! When it is not practical to follow the entire plan, don't sweat it. Just jump back in the groove when you get home. Remember that the entire point of this is to improve your quality of life!

WHAT TO EXPECT

You may not understand all the details of how each habit works, and that is okay. My goal in the following chapters is to earn your trust enough to get you to try. If you implement these habits consistently, they can change your body within a very short period.

In fact, my parents changed so much—in a good way—and so quickly that I was personally shocked. I did not expect that they would achieve such an extreme positive change. They could not have been more pleased with their new level of increased energy, the way they felt, and the way they looked. And learning that their blood work showed such drastic improvements further confirmed that this was *real* change.

You should know that my parents followed this plan to the letter in those first three months. They were not trying, they were doing, and they are still reaping the rewards of their effort.

I share the concepts contained here in bits and pieces all day long every day with my patients, depending on their needs at that time. This is the first time I have put this information together in a way that anyone can easily read, understand, implement, and use as a lifelong reference.

At the end of each chapter, I give you action steps so you can easily implement the habit into your life, followed by a recap of why that habit is important.

You will also see my website www.ChrisPerron.com referenced, at times, as a resource. The content in this book has stood the test of time but how to accomplish the goals will continue to evolve and my website is the most efficient way to share the most up-to-date advice and is recommended as a supplemental resource.

CAN I ADOPT JUST ONE OR TWO OF THE HABITS?

These 7 Habits for Healthy Living that I'm teaching you are meant to be done as a group. But allow me to clarify: each of the habits, if implemented, will contribute to your overall health. However, if done as a group, they will work in coordination with each other and exponentially improve your health. The entire basis of The Simple Plan is that you need *all* seven habits if you want to be healthy. Any one of the habits, if not implemented, will put a drag on the overall improvement. Imagine if someone was 400 pounds and then they implemented something that brought them to 300 pounds, but that was their new plateau. Yes, it's technically "good" that they dropped weight, but they are still obese and likely to have a heart attack, etc. Therefore, to really get the entire benefit, *you need all seven habits.* That is actually the magic of the plan.

Let's look at eating, for instance, which I'll cover in Simple Habit 3. Certainly, what we eat on a daily basis is absolutely one of the primary things that you should do on purpose and begin to improve as soon as possible. Eating well can be a monumental shift for you and may initially be one of the hardest habits to transition to. It does require several steps as well as new knowledge and skills.

I am telling you this to be up-front with what to expect. I also want you to cut yourself some slack. Make this a transition, because realistically that is the only way to do this. Some aspects of eating better are straightforward, but finding your groove may take a little time and that is normal. Progress is the goal; perfection is not real. Wherever you are starting from, is what it is. Recognize that, accept it, and then start the transition.

WHY FOLLOW MY METHOD?

Aside from the fact that my parents experienced astonishing success following my simple suggestions, you may be wondering what led me to chiropractic, and how I've seen these habits work for others.

In a story I'll describe in more detail later in the book, I had to reorient my path after a failed bid to go to the United States Naval Academy. Since that path was no longer an option, I accepted an Army ROTC scholarship to be an electrical engineer major at the University of Miami. This was quite the honor as well and although it was not my dream of being a Navy SEAL, I was good in math and science so engineering was the logical next best path. However, I had no actual idea what an engineer did. Within a few weeks of classes I had already determined that I was bored out of my mind and not interested in doing what I was being taught for the next forty years of my life. I "majored" in the crew team and loved my ROTC class, where I got an A, but unfortunately earned far lower grades in the classes more important to my major.

I left Miami and the scholarship after one year. I enrolled in Northern Virginia Community College. While I was away my freshman year, my mother had taken a job with some local chiropractors. As a benefit to her, we were able to be treated for free. As an eighteen-year-old, I found it fun and interesting. I was also at a crossroads of thinking about the path I wanted to take. Then entered Dr. Andy Smith, my first chiropractor. He was full of energy and relatively fresh out of school. He said, "Why don't you become a chiropractor? You can help lots of people, make a good living, and retire young." That was the literal pitch, and to an eighteen-year-old, that is quite the pitch. I look back and think how thankful I am for things working out as well as they have. I love being a chiropractor and helping people.

I looked up what the requirements were for attending chiropractic school and discovered that it was the same as pre-med. That means a lot of science classes. I enrolled in several classes at the community college to start to pile up the prerequisites. At Northern Virginia Community College, they required the students to meet with a guidance counselor to review their courses for enrollment. I met with mine and she looked at my course selection and said, "You can't take these." I asked, "Why not?" She said that it would be too hard. I asked if *I* was allowed to take them, or did *she* have that control? She said that I could make the decision, but she was strongly advising against my course selection. Of course, I did it anyway and earned all As and a B. That was a lesson in the fact that when you go after something you want, the effort is secondary. Everything you do takes effort; channel it towards fueling the life you want.

One of the keys in life is identifying what you enjoy and are good at and then striving to incorporate more of that into your life. You are likely capable of doing many things, but identifying which of those things you have a passion for is where you'll find your personal fulfillment sweet spot.

My ambitious approach to school allowed me to earn my doctorate degree by the age of twenty-three. I became a master of my chosen technique, Activator Methods Chiropractic Technique, and was offered a teaching position by the age of twenty-eight. This honor placed me into an inner circle of chiropractors with decades of experience from whom I soaked up knowledge like a sponge. I have owned and operated one of the top practices in the country for twenty-six years and was named "Virginia Chiropractor of the Year" in 2021, by the Virginia Chiropractic Association.

I have been told that I have a gift for communicating complex information in simple terms to help people understand and therefore utilize the information. As a bonus, I like to keep things light and have fun. I figure the information is the same either way, but the attitude and mood we bring to it is a choice. And I heard somewhere that "laughter is the best medicine."

That is enough about me; this book is about you.

Are you ready to make your own positive changes? Then follow me to the first healthy habit.

INCORPORATE CHIROPRACTIC!

*"Medicine is the study of disease and what causes man to die.
Chiropractic is the study of health and what causes man to live."*

—B.J. PALMER

CAITLYN JENNER (FORMERLY BRUCE JENNER)

The US Olympic Team was preparing for the 1976 Summer Olympics in Montreal. The most famous athlete from the 1976 Summer Olympics was none other than Bruce Jenner. Currently, better known as Caitlyn Jenner. That is right, kids. When Caitlyn was a young Bruce, she won the gold medal in the men's decathlon. Bruce was the best track and field athlete of his time.

Leading into the Montreal Olympics, the US Olympic Committee was deciding which support staff would be part of the team. Dr. Leroy R. Perry, a Los Angeles chiropractor who had worked with Bruce and several other Olympians, did not make the cut to be part of the support staff that would go to Montreal to care for the athletes during the Olympic games. That is, until Bruce Jenner and several of the other top track and field athletes demanded that Dr. Perry be part of the team. They had experienced and understood the value of chiropractic and knew if they were to be at their best, they would need to make sure that their structure and function were also at their best. Dr. Perry ended up being included on the staff and, as the saying goes...the rest is history.

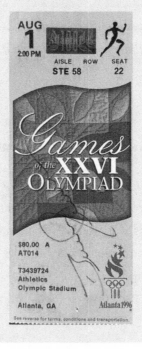

Three weeks after earning my Doctor of Chiropractic degree, I had the privilege of meeting Bruce Jenner at the 1996 Summer Olympics in Atlanta. I was working as a host to top executives for corporate sponsor, International Paper, which involved such strenuous activities as hanging out in a luxury suite at the track and field stadium on the evening Michael Johnson racked up a gold medal in the 200-meter dash. The luxury suite next to us was occupied by Visa who had apparently invited prior gold medal winning decathletes, Bruce Jenner and Bob Mathias. When I caught sight of Bruce, I left our suite and went next door. Since we were already past the serious security I was able to walk right over and have a chat with Bruce! I had him autograph my ticket stub to memorialize the experience. He was a gracious and friendly person and had a strong connection to chiropractic.

WHY CHIROPRACTIC?

I am a chiropractor and have enjoyed helping people for twenty-six years and counting. You're probably not surprised that chiropractic care is the first habit in this plan. Stick with me for a moment as I explain. There is a good reason why this is the starting point for improving your health. Did you know that chiropractic care, and what it offers, impacts every single function that takes place in the human body?

You are right that neck and back pain are the two most

common reasons why people come to see a chiropractor. Thankfully, most of the time, chiropractic care is effective for your neck and back pain.

The reason why we can help people with neck and back pain is because the pain is often the result of structural issues in the spine and other areas of the skeleton. Your skeleton and your nervous system respond to your joints being out of place and stuck.

When a joint gets shifted and stuck far enough out of place that your body cannot self-correct, your brain kicks into high gear to compensate as a survival mechanism. First, your muscles grab on tight and try to pull the joint back into its proper position, but in this situation, called a subluxation, it's too stuck, and it won't realign. As your muscles do that, you might experience a muscle spasm, as your muscles contract and don't relax, which can be painful. Then, as time goes on, your brain realizes that the joint is just too stuck for your muscles to correct its position. Your brain decides it must move on to Plan B.

Plan B is your muscles continuing to hold on tight to the joint to brace it. That's how your body tries to stop the problem from getting worse. Then, the body begins to create compensating patterns. We all will experience this at some point, to various degrees. The longer that your body uses compensating patterns, the more your body will get used to using those patterns. Those patterns are not how your body is supposed to work. They're a way to cope with a joint being out of position, negatively impacting your muscles and nerves. The compensating patterns are a compromise, and your health is not ideal when your body makes compromises.

These compromises—the compensating patterns of the muscles and misaligned joints—have an impact on your nervous system. Think about your knees, ankles, elbows, shoulders, and spine. These are joints that chiropractors work on every day. And we get great results by helping to release the fixation to allow the joints to regain their proper position and function. But while a bone is in the wrong place, they are a burden on your brain and nervous system. It is like having a fire going that your body is constantly trying to keep at bay. At a minimum, it will be an annoyance and a distraction. It can also be extreme enough to where you can't walk, have a migraine, or experience any other type of system malfunction also known as "disease."

Now let's get to the center of it all, your central nervous system, which is your spinal cord and brain. That's where the biggest impacts can take place. Your spine is made up of twenty-four movable vertebrae. In between each one of those movable vertebrae, two nerves exit off your spinal cord, one nerve to the left and one to the right. When you are healthy and your body is properly aligned, those nerves are free to go about their business and communicate information clearly from your body parts to your brain, and from your brain to your body parts. It's a constant information feedback cycle so that your brain can properly coordinate the functions of your entire body, down to each and every cell.

The good news is that we do not have to stay in this compromised state. *That's the whole point of chiropractic.*

CHIROPRACTIC BEST PRACTICES
BABY MARY

A young mother brought her newborn daughter, Mary, in one day for me to evaluate her and see what I might be able to do. I love taking care of babies! What a gift to be able to support the health of a baby to grow and develop without the burden of compensating patterns.

I walked into the exam room to see the most beautiful baby. Blue eyes, perfectly round big cheeks, and a great smile... you know, just like the Gerber baby along with the baby smell and a hint of vanilla. At first look, I assumed this was more of a "well baby" visit, which is great. Just take a moment to check and see if there is any room for improvement or simply confirm she is as perfect as she seems.

Then Mary's mom slid off her little pink fluffy jacket and revealed her right arm that was completely twisted. The entire arm from the shoulder socket was turned as far as you could turn your arm and that is how it stayed. I asked, "Did something happen to create this or was Mary born this way?" The mom confirmed that Mary was born this way. She went on to relay that she had consulted with several top doctors in the area and that the consensus recommendation was to break Mary's upper arm, turn the lower half to where they believed straight to be and reattach it.

This is one of those moments where my outside voice says, "Okaaay." While my inside voice is saying, "Holy sh#$!" I could not imagine this beautiful little girl going through such a procedure and she would still be left with a twisted shoulder. I thought of Mary's life. Sports? Probably not. Playing with the other kids and doing all that everyone else is doing? Probably not. Early arthritis and a lifetime of compensating and dealing with this? Probably.

I asked if there had been any anatomical reason for her arm being this way that was found through the X-rays and other tests that were done. She said there was not, just that her arm was severely twisted.

I asked her to lay Mary on the exam table and I performed an evaluation through the Activator Methods Chiropractic Technique. This is a gentle technique that I have specialized in throughout my entire career. It is extremely precise in the analysis and just as effective in the treatment with the use of the Activator adjusting instrument. There is no twisting or cracking involved, just a quick tap from the instrument that feels like someone tapping you with their finger. I use this technique for precision, but most of my patients love that it is also gentle. At the end of this chapter, there is a link to a demonstration video on my YouTube channel to show you how it works.

Upon evaluation, I found several problems related to Mary's arm. I knew that I could not hurt Mary with my treatment, so it was help or nothing. Mary's mom gave me the go ahead to treat her. It only took a minute to do all that I could. Immediately, Mary started to move her arm a little more than she had previously, but I did not get my hopes up too much. Significant change is rarely immediate. I told Mary's mom to bring her back the next day, so I could evaluate her again and check her response to treatment.

I do not overpromise, as that does not help anyone. I explained that my tests would tell me if Mary's joints were restricted in a way that I could help. If my evaluation showed there was nothing more I could do, I would see what that translated to, with regard to how twisted her arm was, and go from there. Clearly the proposed surgery was not desirable and postponing it a week or so would not negatively affect Mary.

The next day, Mary and her mom came in, and this time

Mary's mom had the biggest smile. She pulled off Mary's pink fluffy jacket to reveal Mary's arm. Her arm was almost normal! My eyes welled up as I got to reimagine Mary's life. She would never even know this had been an issue. Only through a wild story her mom could tell her, as I am sharing with you now.

With a couple more treatments, in the same week, Mary's arm completely released and was perfect, like the rest of her. I could tell you about many other success stories. Like the twins whose heads were stuck tilted, one to the left and one to the right. Just the way they were likely crammed in their mother's womb when space got tight. We got the same results for them as for Mary.

CLEAR PATHWAYS AHEAD

The term for Mary's condition is called a subluxation. Chiropractic is all about finding and evaluating misalignments that are causing strain on your muscles, overall nervous system, and skeleton, and then setting you free. By correcting the subluxation, we release the burden on your body, including any impact on the nerves. It's like a bad phone or internet connection that's choppy and cutting in and out. Your brain gets *some* of the information that your body is sending to it, but your brain is not getting *all* the information. Our body parts are trying to report what's going on, and what they need. But when there's a subluxation interfering with that communication, a chiropractic adjustment can help to clear up that connection, clear up the communication, and help your brain to get the full and correct information from your body parts, so your brain can do what it's made to do. It's made to coordinate your body's functions.

This is why chiropractic care is the centerpiece of everything else, and why I start with it as the first Simple Habit in improving your health. If your structure and function are compromised, you can't be as healthy as you otherwise could be.

Think of it this way: you can eat nutritious food, and that would be helpful. But if your body doesn't know what to do with those nutrients—because the information about the nutrients isn't getting passed between your brain and your body properly—that food is not going to be as helpful to your body and therefore won't improve your health.

Maybe you can't sleep because you're in pain. Maybe you can't sleep because your nervous system is bombarded with distractions from bones that are slightly out of position, and your body can't get into a state of rest and let you sleep, literally.

Maybe you can't exercise because you're in pain. If you're in pain, that's your body saying, "Please don't do that." Where does that leave you? You can't exercise.

What about the impact on your mindset if you're in pain, sleep deprived, and inactive? I can tell you that if I was in pain, couldn't sleep, and my body was agitated and irritated, my mood wouldn't be the best.

FINDING A GOOD CHIROPRACTOR

At my office, Perron Chiropractic, in Reston, Virginia, we treat patients from all over the world. We are ten minutes from Dulles International Airport and patients have had their friends and family come from Africa, Europe, Asia, and throughout the United States for evaluation and treatment. Most of our patients come from all over the Washington, DC, metro area. I am flattered by their trust, demonstrated in their effort to be seen, and honor that trust by always doing my best by them. But what if you do not live near Washington, DC, or have the ability or desire to come to town for an extended visit?

How do you know if your chiropractor is doing a good job for your needs? I emphasize *your needs*. There are many chiropractic techniques and all are good for some things and none are good for everything. My advice has always been to go with the results, including to my patients wondering if I am the right fit for them. Before you see your chiropractor, decide what your personal definition of success is for your time, effort, and expense and then share that with them.

If your chiropractor responds in any way other than supportive and then with a game plan of what they believe they can and maybe cannot do to help you achieve *your goal*, that might be a red flag. Your goal should be the only goal that matters, not theirs. We are also not miracle workers, so your goal may not be realistic in our opinion and we should be able to explain why and maybe reframe your goal to something that is more realistic. Open and honest communication is paramount and that needs to come from both parties, the doctor and you.

I am often asked the understandable question of how long it should take to get results or how many visits to fix you. Unfortunately, there is no answer to give you. You are an individual with your own life history that has brought you to this point in time. You also have your own ongoing habits and patterns that may be bad or good. There are a lot of factors that determine your level of success and how quickly you may achieve it. This is why I would focus on finding a chiropractor whom you trust and then trusting that doctor. This should include the chiropractor's opinion on what your expectations should be. Then, do your part by following instructions and, by all means, hold your doctor to their part of meeting those expectations.

Here are some helpful resources in narrowing your search for a good chiropractor near you.

To find a doctor who is properly trained in the Activator Methods Chiropractic Technique, go to www.activator.com and use their "Find A Doc" tool to find someone near you. I only recommend "Advanced Proficiency Rated" or "Instructors." Avoid "Proficiency," not because they are bad, but they are not yet trained to the level that would make them special with the Activator Methods Chiropractic Technique.

Activator Methods Chiropractic Technique Demo Video can be viewed on my website:

www.ChrisPerron.com

*This is a specialty and there may not be anyone near you that is practical.

There are plenty of good chiropractors using other techniques as well. Here are a couple of things to look for that may help in your search.

Are they members of their state association? We have the Unified Virginia Chiropractic Association in Virginia and every state has their own as well and typically a "Find A Doc" search tool. Why does belonging to a state association mean anything? It shows that he or she is likely to be up to date on everything going on in the chiropractic profession and the kind of person who wants to be informed and keep up with best practices. I was president of the Unified Virginia Chiropractic Association from 2019 to 2021 and can attest that in Virginia the members work hard to be their best for their patients.

Last but not least, check Google reviews. That's right. What are other people saying? If there are a lot of happy patients willing to take a minute to share their story for your benefit, that says something. I have found Google reviews to be the best reflection of reality. I have found Yelp to not be as accurate. Different algorithms garner different results for what makes it online.

These are general suggestions on how you might narrow your search. The main thing is to pick one and figure it out firsthand.

ACTION STEPS:

☐ Write down your definition of success as you see things right now. Don't worry about what you think is realistic or not; make your wish list. Example: I would like to be pain free, fully functional, and have some knowledge on what I can do to sustain that level of health.

☐ Have this conversation with your chiropractor to make sure you are both on the same page. We are not mind readers. This can help us to help you.

☐ If you currently don't have a chiropractor, get one. Use the tips above to get started. You must include this foundational habit of The Simple Plan.

RECAP: WHY CHIROPRACTIC?

Let's take that scenario I mentioned above about being in pain, sleep deprived, and inactive and turn it around. Let us take the burden of irritation or pain off your nervous system and get rid of those distractions. You would begin to function better, you could exercise, and you could rest better. How would that affect your mindset and outlook on life? You can easily see how these different pieces tie together. Bruce "Caitlyn" Jenner, Baby Mary's mom, and countless others can attest to the power of chiropractic care. Including chiropractic as the foundation of The Simple Plan establishes a firm base upon which you can establish all of the other simple habits. Correcting subluxations allows your body to have clear communication with your brain, which can clear the way for numerous health improvements. Just as I "reset" my mom with a chiropractic adjustment after her heart attack, we can all use a reset from time to time or when a more complicated issue arises.

RESTORE YOUR GUT AND BRAIN

"All disease begins in the gut."

—HIPPOCRATES

TOMMY TOLD US: A TRUE STORY

One day, a wonderful, friendly family of a mom, teenage daughter, and younger son came into the office for a "checkup." The son is autistic and nonverbal, and such a sweet kid, whom I will call Tommy. My day is always brighter when they come in. It had been many months since I had last seen them, which was not unusual. The primary patient on this day was Tommy. I am always curious about my patient's perspectives, so I asked the mom, "How do you know when to bring him?"

"He told us."

I was astonished. "What?"

Then she told me about *The Nemechek Protocol*. I looked it up that day and ordered the book by the same title. By the end of the week, I had finished reading it, and I was sold enough to try this protocol with my own family. I had been searching for over a decade to the tune of tens of thousands of dollars, a lot of effort, even more frustration, and little progress to show for it for gut issues in my own house.

I had heard many concepts, and tried many protocols that made sense on paper, but in practice they produced little or no noticeable benefit. Now, I had the simplest protocol I had ever seen, an increased understanding of the science behind it, and a firsthand account of Tommy, who was greatly benefiting from following the protocol. It was worth a try.

GUT AND BRAIN RESTORATION BASICS

As you will read in the next chapter on food, there are ways to treat your body better, especially the gut that has the primary interaction with everything you consume. To be blunt, food alone may take another lifetime to achieve getting your gut back in order. You may be the exception but I would not bank on it. Therefore, this habit, which is front-end focused, can restore your gut to a healthy state. Then, the next five habits will help you to sustain. I recommend doing the Gut and Brain Restoration Program at least once for anyone who is serious about being their best. It is a fast track to getting your gut working at its best for you.

HOW DO YOU KNOW IF YOU NEED THIS?

Any digestive issues, bloating, food sensitivities, constipation, diarrhea, or any other conditions that translate to "your gut is malfunctioning"? Have you ever had an antibiotic? Periods of sustained stress? Eat fast food? Drink soda? Do a lot of your meals come in a portable container? Are you overweight? Do you get my point?

To be clear, the Gut and Brain Restoration Program, like The Simple Plan as a whole, cures nothing and treats no disease. The aim is to make you healthier and provide your body a better chance of cleaning up its own messes, as it is designed to do.

GUT AND BRAIN RESTORATION PROGRAM

The program is meant to be a ninety day reset, not a long-term crutch. The program is ideally designed to work towards getting you ahead of the curve where sustaining good health is practical through the other habits. With that said, there is only one way to incorporate this habit and that is through a specific supplement protocol. No way around it.

I derived part of the Gut and Brain Restoration Program from *The Nemechek Protocol* by Dr. Nemechek. His book is an excellent resource if you want to learn more about gut-brain interactions.

The synopsis of Dr. Nemechek's protocol is to begin by taking an antibiotic that blasts out all the bacteria in the gut, good and bad, as it is impossible for an antibiotic to differentiate. I was not so keen on that piece. That is why I switched for my Gut Restoration Program. I believe it is a better approach, since it addresses the bad bacteria while simultaneously bolstering the good bacteria. It does not use any antibiotics, since they cause damage to the good bacteria as well.

I agree with Dr. Nemechek on what you should do next and keep doing for the long run. And it's simple, since you only need to do three easy things:

1. Take good quality omega-3 DHA supplements to support the microglia in your brain. This helps them to do their job of pruning the neural pathways.
2. Consume at least an ounce of organic extra virgin olive oil (OEVOO) each day. Consuming the OEVOO is the key, and I recommend that you eat it with food, such as in salad dressing, cooking, or baking with it. But some palm and canola oil allows some latitude in what you consume.
3. Avoid consuming all oils other than OEVOO, palm oil, and canola oil. Try to keep the canola to a minimum or

none. I know there are other oils that are probably fine and canola is not very popular but my goal is to keep it simple. Simple is OEVOO.

90 DAY SUPPLEMENTATION

Here is a simple outline of which supplements you need to take at each stage of the 90 Day Gut and Brain Restoration Program.

THE BASIC 90 DAY GUT AND BRAIN RESTORATION PROGRAM

Days 1-30	
MegaSpores	2/day with food
IgG2000	2/day with food
DHA (Omega-3)	4,000mg/day

Days 31-60	
MegaSpores	2/day with food
HU58	2/day with food
MegaPrebiotic	1 scoop/day
DHA (Omega-3)	4,000 mg/day

Days 61-90	
MegaSpores	2/day with food
MegaPrebiotic	1 scoop/day
MegaMucosa	1 scoop/day
DHA (Omega 3)	4,000 mg/day

In the recap, I'll share where you can get these supplements and more information on the program itself. You don't need to be my patient to qualify for the program.

ALL ILLNESS BEGINS IN THE GUT

Have you ever taken antibiotics, eaten processed food, or been under stress?

Of course. We all have.

Do you have any noticeable digestive challenges? (reflux, constipation, stomach upset, frequent diarrhea, bowel movements less than once a day, food sensitivities, brain fog, focus issues, etc.) If so, you really want to pay attention.

The truth is that your gut takes a beating over your lifetime and to an extent it is built for it. However, antibiotics and processed food were not part of the natural equation and stress continues to skyrocket over recent decades.

This Simple Habit is about acknowledging and accepting what I just stated as fact and then doing something about it. Taking one pill after the next to dampen symptoms is not the answer. It is pretending everything is okay, merely covering symptoms, all while your gut digs a deeper hole for you to suffer the effects of later.

What I will describe to you here is a simple process that is like the concept of chiropractic. The Gut and Brain Restoration Program and chiropractic are about repairing the damage that has been done. The goal is getting you as close to a clean slate as possible and then the remaining five habits are about staying well by reinforcing the positive.

LEAKY GUT SYNDROME

The gut wall is supposed to be a barrier to toxins while also drawing in the nutrients that we need. So, what is leaking?

When the gut "leaks," the toxins are getting through. The longer your body stays in this state, the more damage the toxins create. It is like having several holes in a boat. Would you simply treat the resultant water damage and work on bailing out the water that is getting through the hull? Of course not. The first thing you need to do is to fix the leaks; otherwise, your other efforts will be futile, and any progress will be short lived.

This is common sense with a boat, but why is this thought process so foreign when it comes to your body? Take this pill for that symptom and this pill for another symptom and then this pill for the side effects of the other pills, and so on. Mind boggling!

My recommendation is that you begin to shift your thinking from "symptom free equals healthy" to "healthy equals healthy." An easy example is pain medication. You take enough and your pain will go away, but will that make you healthy? Of course not.

Let's keep working on the foundation of your health where many of the causes of disease can be found, then shore up your foundation, and "magically" many symptoms go away. Why? People in a state of health don't have symptoms.

WHAT ABOUT THE BRAIN?

Toxins can make it hard for your brain to do its normal process of "pruning." Our brains never stop growing and building new neural pathways, like a garden that's always growing. What happens if you never weed or prune the bushes? That's right, they become a mess of branches and roots going every which way with no clear path. Remember Mr. Miyagi in the movie *Karate Kid*, as he meticulously pruned his Bonsai trees? In our brains, the caretakers of our neural gardens are called microglia, and they can be impeded by the toxins stemming from a Leaky Gut.

The Gut and Brain Restoration Program aims to restore the correct balance of healthy bacteria in your gut so they can absorb nutrients and fill in the leaks that have been overrun by the bad bacteria. The good bacteria mend the leaks.

In this scientifically proven program, we accomplish this by feeding the good bacteria to promote their growth. At the same time, the good bacteria "marks" the bad bacteria in a way that triggers your immune system to come and get rid of them. By promoting the good bacteria and eliminating the bad bacteria, the gut steadily repairs itself. Like fertilizing your lawn, the bare patches steadily fill back in and the weeds get overrun by healthy grass when supported correctly.

FOOD MATTERS

The food you eat and the beverages you drink have a significant impact on your health. Good food and beverages reinforce a healthy gut and provide the nutrients your body needs to take care of itself. Bad food and beverages cause damage to the gut and can lead to it creating leaks. Bad food is like having an NFL game played on your lawn. It might be fun in the moment, but what a mess after it's done. The next Simple Habit will explain healthy eating and how to make it easy.

It's important to support your brain's health, too. As I shared, a gut that is leaking toxins can hurt your brain. Fixing those leaks by following the simple 90 Day Gut and Brain Restoration Program is vital, and you can also support your brain by supplementing omega-3 fatty acids. It's simple if you take good quality supplements, especially with high amounts of DHA.

ACTION STEPS:

- ☐ Start using only organic extra virgin olive oil (OEVOO) in your home.
- ☐ Take a high-quality omega-3 supplement daily. Nordic Naturals DHA 1000 is what I prescribe to my patients. (Adults) 2/day for sustaining health, 4/day if trying to improve your health.
  *As always, check with your doctor.
- ☐ Enroll in the Gut and Brain Restoration Program—www. ChrisPerron.com.

RECAP: WHY RESTORE THE GUT AND BRAIN?

The gut is one place where I recommend you simply pay the piper and do it. Acknowledge reality and that this is the likely fastest path to a healthier gut.

The fact is that to the extent your gut is a leaking ship, or a torn up lawn, it will continuously wreak havoc on your health even if you are doing all good things currently. Bite the bullet, and invest the time and effort in yourself. Do the program, and get on with your life!

FEED YOUR BODY

"When diet is wrong, medicine is of no use. When diet is correct, medicine is of no use."

—AYURVEDIC PROVERB

EAT LIKE THE QUEEN

In September 1984, Queen Elizabeth II walked up to me to say hello. I was standing with the rest of my class fifty meters from the front doors of the Canadian Parliament Buildings. It was a sunny day, and the temperature was in the sixties. People were lined up on either side of the promenade to greet the queen for her royal visit and my class won the lottery at my school and got the prize of this field trip. Just being in the crowd instead of English class would have been enough of a prize. But instead we were positioned right up front on the left heading toward the Parliament Buildings and Queen Elizabeth II decided to stop for a moment right where I was standing. The amusing irony is that she stopped at the American kid. My father was an officer in the US Army and our family was stationed in Ottawa, Canada (the nation's capital), for three years as a part of a NATO exchange program.

Queen Elizabeth II shared some pleasantries with my friends and me. She commented that I looked tall and healthy and that I must be eating my vegetables. I responded with, "Yes, ma'am." Obviously, it was a pretty surreal moment that makes for a good story later, but in preparing for writing this book I recalled this conversation and researched the queen's eating habits, since clearly she must be doing something right. As it turns out she practices what she preaches. She eats fairly simply. Plenty of fresh vegetables, fish, and lean meats. Always fresh and high quality but not "rich" foods or processed foods. Her main vice is chocolate cake. But generally she keeps a routine and eats simple and healthy food. Her health and longevity is an example to emulate. My recommendation is...to eat like the queen!

LEARN TO FISH

I mean that figuratively from the saying: *Give a man a fish and he eats for a day, teach him to fish and he eats for a lifetime.*

My goal for you when it comes to food is to teach you to

"fish." Translated...make your own food! It is the only way to eat healthy, unless you have the funds to have a private chef, and that would work, too. Just hand them this book and ask them to work in this space. The reason most diets don't work is that they are extreme or at least cumbersome and you could never sustain them for the long term. When you stop, everything reverts back because you only learned to be extreme or take on a part-time job of counting points or calories. Ugh! Other weight loss programs may have you continually purchase their food and some may even be relatively healthy meals but it is all about portion control. So it is not only expensive but you are still hungry. That, too, can get old and expensive after a while and, again, you never learned anything to sustain yourself. The Simple Plan pulls the curtain back from the kitchen and makes eating healthy and attainable for the long term. I love to eat! What I will share is my eating regimen that I shared with my parents. It was the primary source of their weight loss and improved health. All seven habits combine to support one another but this is where it is at for the biggest impact for sustained great results.

Open your mind and follow along as I reveal to you what is possible, and yet simple.

THE MEDITERRANEAN DIET

My daughter Becca's dance company (Encore Performers)

was performing in Italy for a couple of weeks in the summer of 2018, and my son, parents, and I were excited to follow the tour as groupies. One afternoon, my son Matthew and I were enjoying Monterosso al Mare, a small seaside village on the Mediterranean. The region is called Cinque Terre after its five small fishing villages. Cinque Terre's trademark is the landscape of colorful buildings cascading down hillsides to the water. The sky was bright blue with a couple of puffy white clouds, and we had been swimming at the beach. We took a break and walked a block along a cobblestone street to find a restaurant to have lunch.

We decided on spaghetti Bolognese, a classic Italian meal to help us fully experience being in Italy. It was everything I had hoped for—it was fresh, it was delicious, and the village scenery seemed to amplify its flavors. A perfect moment in my life.

I'm sharing this experience with you because the healthiest diet has been shown to be the Mediterranean diet, and we were gobbling that diet up with a lot of enthusiasm.

A Mediterranean diet is based on a lot of fresh vegetables, fish, lean meats, some fruit, and plenty of olive oil. In particular, extra virgin olive oil. This simple basic foundation for meals in the Mediterranean region is full of nutrients. It has everything that we need, and there's really not much of anything that we don't need. Whether your taste buds would prefer to take you to Greece, Italy, France, Spain, or even Morocco, you're guaranteed to find plenty of great meal options that will satisfy your appetite.

There are almost endless options for how to make your food. That's one of the big keys because if you're currently not much of a cook, don't shy away from this simple approach to eating. It does not have to be complex. In fact, if you aren't much of a cook, you simply may not have been exposed to or experienced cooking. I want you to know that a Mediterranean diet is only as hard as you want to make it, and it's as easy as you want it to be, too.

COOKING AND SALAD OILS

One key is using the right kind of oil. We talked about organic EVOO, which is the main oil used in the Mediterranean, and a couple of other options. When buying salad dressings, read the label! Even organic dressings rarely use EVOO; most use soybean oil because it is cheaper and can also be "organic," but that does not make it good for you.

Look up recipes online on how to make your own. It is easier than you think.

FAST AND EASY FOOD

The sky's the limit when it comes to cooking! When it

comes to the Mediterranean region of the world, cooking can be a very simple task. For ideas and inspiration, you can use the internet or YouTube, and there are even on-demand courses that teach cooking. For cooking lessons on demand, you just need to buy the ingredients and follow along with the chef. I include cooking videos in my private coaching programs as well that walk you through how to make some of my favorite recipes. We will walk you through the motions of learning to cook. It can be healthy for you and tasty, too. And it might just be fun!

EASY EATING AT HOME

Eating at home is vital because it is almost impossible to eat healthy on a regular basis and eat out on a regular basis. Why is that?

You might find a rare restaurant that uses ingredients as healthy and as pure as you would buy for making your own meals at home. At a restaurant, the challenge is they have to operate with a profit margin to earn a living. Things like low-cost soybean oil are extremely popular in the restaurant industry and those ingredients are terrible for your health.

If a restaurant uses extra virgin olive oil (EVOO), it's usually highlighted on the menu because they want you to know about it. If you don't see it, and you rarely will unless it's a higher end or health food restaurant, then just know that what you're eating is not going to be nearly as healthy as a meal you could make at home.

EATING OUT

Does this mean you can never eat out? A restaurant experience can be fantastic. I certainly enjoy it. But for the maximum health benefit, eating out needs to follow the 95:5 rule.

Eat at home most of the time (95 percent of the time). Eating out should be the exception to the rule. It should happen in a pinch, it should be on a special occasion, but it should not be your normal routine. It is easy to get into a routine of just popping through the drive-through. I know because I have lived it, too. It is all about your habits. One of mine was getting in the groove on a daily basis where my truck just headed to Chick-Fil-A at lunchtime, or worse when I used to find myself there at breakfast time, too, after dropping the kids off at school. The chicken breakfast burritos are killer! And the waffle fries...don't get me started. It's easy for all of us to get caught up in a mindless habit. In today's busy world, we have so much to think about and keep track of that the convenience of quick food is all too enticing. We fall into the trap of sacrificing our health in the name of perceived efficiency. I say "perceived" because eating poorly actually drags down your energy, creating more frequent, time-consuming, and financially costly issues. You really are not being efficient when you hit the drive-through, you are being short-sighted. Quickly your routines turn into autopilot, and usually stay that way until there is a problem.

SECRET WEAPON: THE SMOOTHIE

The smoothie for lunch, especially during the 90 Day Transformation, is strongly recommended; in fact, I would say required for best results. Not just any smoothie though. Most smoothie shops have lots of sugar added to make them taste good while making you think it is healthy for you. Or smoothies that are all fruit and fruit juice, so again they are sweet, but we are not meant to ingest two mangoes, three oranges, a pint of blueberries, a banana, and ten strawberries all at once. This is too much sugar! Even if the source is good.

My recipe that all who have tried have liked is:

½ cup organic orange juice

1 scoop Vega One meal replacement (Coconut Almond flavor)

1 medium-size banana

roughly 1 cup ice cubes

¼ cup filtered water

Put it all in a blender and hit the switch!

It's that simple. I have had this for lunch 95 percent of the time for several years now. I have been 6′ 0″ tall and 196 pounds for most of that time and I have not been hungry, while combined with intermittent fasting (which I will explain later in this chapter). Our bodies want nutrition. This smoothie is packed with nutrition. It is also a major "easy button" in your busy day. My recipe has a bit of a tropical flavor to it. My staff likes the Vega One chocolate flavor with a banana and water. You could use almond or oat milk as a liquid in place of the orange juice. Keep it simple. This will give you one less meal to navigate each day. It is like drinking a multivitamin with protein. You will be saving time, money, and energy. Bottoms up!

FOOD SHOPPING

A big key to eating healthy is the way you shop for your food. My philosophy is if it does not make it in my cart, then it won't make it to my house. If it does not make it in my house, then it won't make it to my mouth. What you have in your house is dangerous. It is the late-night snack, boredom eating, or stress eating that gets us when we are at our weakest. I love many kinds of wine, Ben & Jerry's ice cream, pizza, and Cheez-Its (especially the Extra Toasty ones). You see, it is not a matter of pretending that you don't like what you like. That is a lie you will never be able to sell to yourself and I don't believe you should try to. It only adds stress to pretend. It is the discipline to not buy it, either at all or infrequently. One of the biggest things I do to help this is to do most of my shopping at Whole Foods. Why? They have healthier options to choose from and they don't even sell Cheez-Its! Thank goodness, because it seems that every time I stop in the regular grocery store they are 50 percent off. It is like they knew I was coming! If you are trying not to drink, would you go to a bar on a regular basis? Minimize the temptation.

You want to buy organic food as much as possible. Some foods are more important to stick to organic than others based on farming and production practices. A great resource is the Environmental Working Group at www. ewg.org where they rate food based on pesticides and toxins headlined by their popular list, "The Dirty Dozen." This is a list of the worst foods from a chemical standpoint and foods I suggest not even buying if you can't find them organic. You should check it out at least once. You will likely be surprised—I know I was. A couple of the regulars are strawberries, and really most berries, as well as lettuce of any kind. The extra expense of buying organic is much cheaper than your healthcare expenses in the long run. Look at it as an investment in your most prized possession: you. Also, buy fruits in season. How do you know when they are in season? Simple, they are abundant and often on sale. Supply and demand!

DAIRY

Organic is a must! That is milk, which I don't recommend having as a beverage, and cereal does nothing good for you, so milk should be minimal anyway. Cheese, yogurt, ice cream, and butter are included as well. Yes, I break the rules with my good friends Ben & Jerry occasionally, but if you look at their labels, you can actually read all the words. I was pleasantly surprised as well.

I spent some time with "Jerry" at an event in New York City a couple of years ago and he was such a gracious and genuinely nice guy. He told me that they began and continue to source most of their ingredients from small and local companies. One example is that all the brownies they use in Chocolate Fudge Brownie are made by nuns at a convent! Seriously. Jerry served me some Cherry Garcia that night at a below street-level speakeasy where we were attending a party. My favorite is Chubby Hubby. I love the flavor but I think the messaging in the name keeps me aware to watch out for how often I indulge.

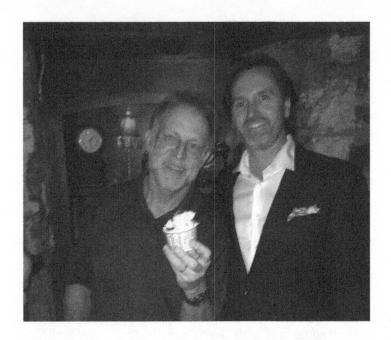

MEAT

"Grass fed" is best. In fact, the nutrient content in grass-fed beef is so much higher than the basic beef that you could eat about half as much and get the same nutrition. Next best is meat "raised with no hormones and no antibiotics." What they pump in cows is toxic to make them much bigger than they would be naturally and then they sell them by the pound. See how that works?

POULTRY

Organic is best. Next best is "raised without hormones or antibiotics." Follow the same rule of thought with eggs.

FISH

Wild caught is best. Why? Fish were meant to swim freely and eat whatever they naturally eat. "Farm raised" fish does not sound right. Try to avoid tilapia, as it is not that healthy and there are so many other choices. Salmon is always good and cod is a great white fish choice, but experiment and figure out what you like.

EXTRA VIRGIN OLIVE OIL (EVOO)

Organic is best. Read the label and stick to olives grown in the United States, Italy, Greece, Spain, or France. Try to stay away from EVOO from other countries, mainly out of being extra cautious about the "organic" oversight.

Last, but not least, you want to shop for *your menu*. Don't go to the store, at least until you get the hang of things, without a shopping list and then stick to the list. Don't get lured by the Cheez-Its sale! Or maybe that's just me.

YOUR MENU

You need to make a house menu.

Now that I have taken you through the rules of the game, I want you to take out a piece of paper and start listing all the meals that you already make and like that fit into the plan. I have found the easiest way to make this shift is to start with what you already know and build from there. Once you have your list, brainstorm, look at cookbooks or websites under Mediterranean Diet, and choose as many additional recipes as needed to get you to at least twelve. Just like at a restaurant, this menu can and should change over time. Your tastes will evolve and you will get bored with certain meals, especially if you eat them too often. Make this a document that is supposed to change with time.

This menu is vital to shifting to this new habit. It is enough mental work to simply do something new. By outlining meals that you enjoy, you can make a shopping list and have clarity when you go to the grocery store. When you get home after work or soccer practice or whatever you do all day and are tired, this system is key. You just look at your menu and choose. You don't start with "What should I eat? I am too tired to figure it out" because suddenly, takeout will appear. You know your schedule best, so you can consider prepping some ingredients in advance so you can just throw things together at the end of your busy day. All of this comes with practice but can become super simple in no time.

INTERMITTENT FASTING

Intermittent fasting has become popular in recent years, but it has been practiced in many cultures for centuries. This is yet another example of research finally catching up with what many have known to be beneficial for a long time.

Intermittent fasting refers to eating on a schedule during a given day. Fasting is choosing not to eat for a certain period of time.

Our bodies love routine! Our bodies thrive on routine!

When our digestive system kicks into gear to digest food and process it to our benefit, it is taxing. It is what our gut is built for, but after working, it also needs a moment to repair and prepare for the next round of food. When you give your gut a lengthy break and you are on a consistent schedule, you are helping provide the time and space for the *repair* and *prepare*. The concept is to allow the gut the time to repair from that day's work. Simply put, to keep pace with the workload. The healthier you eat, combined with the intermittent fasting, the better your gut is able to do what it needs to and keep you functioning at your best.

There are different ways to implement intermittent fasting and a quick search of the internet will reveal endless schedules and rationales. My recommendation is to keep it simple and go with 8 hours on and 16 hours off.

8-HOUR WINDOW

Eat in an 8-hour window each day. The first food item that you eat on a given day starts your clock. I have found that the easiest and most practical approach is to have a window from 11:00 a.m.–7:00 p.m. or 12:00 p.m.–8:00 p.m. Basically...skip breakfast.

What? You may say, *but I was told it was the most important meal of the day!*

Oh, do you mean the bagel, pancakes, or cereal? Just because you were told something does not make it true.

WHAT ABOUT BREAKFAST?

We've all been raised to view breakfast as a vital part of starting the day.

How often do you actually wake up and feel hungry? I don't wake up feeling hungry. When this concept was first shared with me at a professional conference, I discussed it with many of my colleagues and none of them woke up hungry either. We all ate breakfast because we were "supposed to."

Many things in history have been said to be "good" for us—like cigarettes and asbestos to name a couple. An open mind and personal experience are two great learning tools. I started intermittent fasting, or, as I like to call it, intermittent eating, the next day and have not looked back since.

Before you stress any further, coffee does not start your clock. Whew!

Coffee does not mean chemical junk; it means coffee and maybe a splash of organic half and half. Not flavored shots and sugar, and definitely not artificial sweeteners.

For me, what works best is a cup or two of coffee in the morning. No juice and no food.

My 8-hour eating window starts, most days, around 1:00 p.m. That's when I'm usually done with my work for the morning and I most often run home and make myself a smoothie, and that opens my 8-hour eating window. Not everyone has the ability to go home for lunch, depending on where your employment is and where you live. You want to plan ahead and bring your lunch. You will eat better and likely save a lot of money in the process. The point is, you're eating on purpose, and within that 8-hour window only. Not before, and not after the window. Since my window starts around 1:00 p.m., that means my window closes about 9:00 p.m. at night.

I often have snacks in the afternoon that may consist of dates, a piece of fruit, olives, or basically anything you can think of that fits in the food guidelines. Dinner is my main meal of the day and while sticking to the ingredients fitting into the guidelines, I eat all I want.

Many people ask me about portion sizes. This is understandable because a lot of diets are based on portion control. What a hassle to track portions and points. I could never do that personally. This is a big part of this program. Life should not be work! We are just eating. If you are eating within the guidelines above, then eat all you want. You will get tired of chewing and your stomach will tell you it has had enough well before anything bad happens. Do you really think you can get fat on vegetables?

When you are hungry your body is telling you it needs nutrients, it needs fuel. Your body does not crave food; it craves nutrients. Let me repeat that. *Your body does not crave food; it craves nutrients.* This is a vital concept to take in. Why can't we eat just one chip? Because the nutrients are so low that your body says, "Still hungry." So you eat another with the same response from your body and so on. All junk food fits in this category. In fact, some "foods" are negative nutrients. This is when the amount of effort by your body to digest what you ate takes more fuel than the actual food item provided. No wonder you feel tired when you eat poorly. As a bonus, it often stores some of the toxins in the form of fat in your body because there was just too much junk to process and it just could not do it as quickly as you were eating it. That is how we get fat!

I am viewing fat from a health standpoint, not an aesthetic standpoint. Fat is stored toxins! The only healthy way to get rid of it and stay rid of it is to eat healthy, as I have outlined above. Therefore, put few to no toxins in your mouth regularly and you will get all the good stuff you need and allow your body the ability to start working on the backlog of toxins it must process. The intermittent fasting simply adds to providing the time for this work.

The Gut and Brain Restoration Program may be necessary to create an environment where your body is able to take advantage of your healthy eating, as discussed in the previous chapter.

BENEFITS OF ROUTINE

The longer we stay in any routine for our body's sake, physiologically, the more that routine continues to build a benefit upon itself. It is like compound interest. You just get into a groove, and your body will thank you for it.

You may ask, "Does that mean I can never eat anything 'unhealthy' again?" Of course not, but I recommend you start with my 90 Day Transformation Program to kickstart all of the seven habits and exclude all unhealthy things for ninety days. Let me explain further.

MY PROMISE TO YOU...

I can promise you that your taste buds will change. That's one of the coolest things about this process. When you start eating fresh food and eating differently, and taste something you used to love after your taste buds have gotten used to this new way of eating, it's not going to taste the same. In your brain, you'll be thinking something like "Wow, that Big Mac—I haven't had it in a while." I promise you, you'll take one bite of that bad boy, you're going to feel like junk, and you will reevaluate that relationship.

This happened to me several years ago. My family and I were driving overnight to visit my in-laws in Boston, and we left Washington, DC, around midnight. In the rush from work, to packing the car and getting the kids together, I had not eaten dinner and I was starving. I wanted to get going so I figured I would grab something on the way. As it turned out, the only place still open was the McDonald's drive-through. I had not been to a McDonald's in many years but I grew up as a frequent customer. I decided to take a rare walk down this memory lane and ordered my "usual." After that Quarter Pounder with cheese, I wished that I had just starved. My stomach was saying, "What did you do to me?!"

My wish for you is to have a similar experience. Not that I want you to feel bad, but the experience of victory that your physiology has evolved to where it rejects bad things. The reason your body probably does not at the moment is because it is so beaten down that it does not even try. Kind of the same as "building up a tolerance to alcohol." Is that really a goal? That is scary! You know you've made it when your body starts enjoying the good stuff so much that when you give it something that isn't good, your body recognizes it on a chemical level and says, "What are you doing? This is not good."

One thing to be aware of, so that you don't get the wrong idea, is that there are some people who initially experience digestive upset when they begin eating a lot of vegetables. This is often because their bodies are not used to processing healthy food. Please check with your doctor if you have trouble so that he or she can help determine that it is just what I described above versus something that could warrant attention. It is always best to get confirmation that you will be okay. It is amazing to think that you could eat a healthy amount of salad and your body would feel like it's something foreign. That's not where you want to be. If this happens to you, look at it as confirmation that you really need these changes but check in with your doctor to be on the safe side.

I promise you that eating healthy food is amazing. It will likely take a bit of a shift in your skill set, but mostly it is changing your habits. Like every habit, good and bad, the longer you do it, the easier it becomes. The science shows that it takes ninety days to create an autopilot pattern in your brain. It is not a coincidence that this program is a 90 Day Transformation.

The Gut and Brain Restoration Program, outlined in the

previous chapter, is highly recommended for everyone to do at least once, which is why it is a key part of the 90 Day Transformation. Restoring your gut as a launch point to changing your habits can have an exponential impact on your results. Jump in with both feet and achieve your best results, which will only further encourage you to maintain the habits long enough to make them automatic.

We are what we eat. If we are not giving our bodies the nutritional supplies it needs to rebuild, repair, and maintain our health, how can we expect our bodies to build, repair, and maintain our health? Your body is bound to deteriorate. The chemicals you put in your body from modern, processed food is not only bad because of what you're not getting of the good, but you're also actually giving it extra bad to endure. When you eat processed foods, that's a negative; it's not even a neutral.

EATING AND SLEEPING

When you put junk into your body, it affects you on a chemical level. Everything we eat is chemistry. You eat something; it's pulled apart in your intestines to take the good and leave the bad. If your body is getting lots of bad nutrients, and being deprived of good nutrients, that's going to affect your brain as much as anywhere else. When your brain is affected, it can affect your mood, which can affect your attitude, and often your energy level. When your energy level is lower, are you likely to feel like exercising? Probably not. If you are not exercising, will that further decrease your energy level? Of course it will. I think you can see the cycle.

Focus on where you are heading in your health journey, and the direction you are choosing to go. You should not expect that you're just going to flip a switch and do this overnight, particularly if you're not much of a cook right now. Cooking skills can be learned over time. It's not like anybody was born cooking.

I was fortunate that my mother kept a fairly open kitchen, and she did a lot of cooking when I was growing up. I am grateful that, in my childhood, we were fortunate to never be hungry and always had our needs met. But the military doesn't pay a heck of a lot, so we didn't go out a lot either. That was a gift. A gift because my mom was cooking every day and eating out was the exception. I was accustomed to that habit and routine, so I learned to cook at a very young age. I enjoy food. If you enjoy food, it's kind of fun when you can make it yourself because that way you can have what you want, when you want it, how you want it, right? My hope for you is that you'll learn to do this and more importantly, you'll grow to enjoy it. Don't be afraid to try cooking.

ACTION STEPS:

☐ Go through your kitchen and get rid of everything that does not fit what I described.

☐ For the 90 Day Transformation Program, that means no bread, pasta, alcohol, soda, or anything else processed (made for you).

☐ Smoothie for lunch, snack in the afternoon, and dinner. (Tip: Vega ONE's best pricing is typically online.)

☐ Make your menu.

☐ Go grocery shopping for the ingredients for several of the meals on your menu.

☐ Begin intermittent eating. Choose your eight hour eating window and begin.

☐ Decide if you know how to make twelve meals and look into cooking lessons, helpful tips, and further support at www.ChrisPerron.com.

RECAP: WHY HEALTHY FOOD MATTERS

Eating healthy should be enjoyable but you need to first make the shift to better habits. This habit is a process for everyone to varying degrees. Just start moving in the right direction and keep going. Those I have worked with typically comment that it is easier than they expected and tastier than they expected as well. Win, win!

Bon appétit!

SLEEP (PRIORITIZE REST AND RECOVERY)

"Early to bed, early to rise, makes a man healthy, wealthy, and wise."

—BENJAMIN FRANKLIN

UNIVERSITY OF MIAMI CREW TEAM

During my freshman year of college in 1990, I walked on to the crew team at the University of Miami. I played a lot of sports growing up, but this was the first time I had ever seen a crew boat in person. It just looked so cool! Quickly, it became my favorite sport ever. I love the water and watching the sunrise from the intercoastal waterways in Miami was a great combination. I earned the top spot in my boat as the "stroke," setting the pace for the other seven rowers. We were literally the "B" boat heading into the state championships. That meant we were not even considered the best boat on my own team. The weather was stormy and there were waves with whitecaps slamming against the boat. If you have never been in a race boat, the sides are only inches above water level. A boat filled with water is not good for racing. Although I was captain of my high school swim team just the year before, I was not interested in demonstrating that skill set at that time. This was a head race where each boat takes off in a staggered fashion and is timed, so you do not have the ability to know how you are doing relative to the other boats.

In racing there is something called a "power 10" where for ten consecutive strokes everyone rows extra hard. Typically, this is done periodically but it is meant to be a level that can't be sustained for the length of the course. I started to recognize the shoreline as we were rowing and noticed that we were closer to the finish line than anticipated based on how much energy I still had. I told the coxswain to keep calling out "power 10s." At first, he thought I was nuts, but he did what I asked because in the end he knew I was going to do it anyway and everyone sitting behind me just followed my lead. It was only after we finished that we found out that due to the poor conditions, they shortened the racecourse from three miles to two miles.

My boat ended up winning the state championship!

What does rowing have to do with sleep?

Well, practice required me to meet up at the van at 4:30 a.m., six days a week. This was definitely the one negative. When my alarm went off at 4:15 a.m. each day, I had to talk myself into getting up. Every day. I loved rowing, but I hated getting up so early. Still, I would tell myself that I would be happy when I got there and if I didn't go, I would be deprived of the fun. I never missed a practice.

Now, refer back to me being a freshman in college, in Miami! I was apparently pretty good at rowing, but I was also a knucklehead teenager in many ways. For most of my first semester at school, I averaged three to four hours of sleep per night. I also did not have the best nutritional practices. Put it all together and my body finally crashed in the form of "mono." I was sick for a week or so and got past the viral part but I was left with balance issues for months. The bugs made their final stand in my ears and to this day I still have pressure problems if I go more than about six feet below the surface in the water. For someone who loves water, this is a major bummer. And I will let your imagination figure out my GPA for that first semester. Not pretty.

Sleep deprivation, even for a seventeen-year-old collegiate athlete, will get you in the end.

Don't be a teenage knucklehead!

SLEEP IS ESSENTIAL!

Your body does most of its repair and maintenance work while you sleep. When you are deprived of sleep, or when you don't get high-quality sleep, then you're being deprived of that daily or nightly repair work. It is no surprise that people who have poor sleep are going to have poor health. Studies are clear on this fact. When maintenance is missed on an ongoing basis, issues start to pile up. When little problems pile up, do you know what happens? That's right; they become big problems. Sleep is vital, and as simple as it seems to go and lay down, close your eyes, and then open them eight hours later, you may know that it's not always quite that simple.

Here's my advice on sleep. There are some things that you can do directly to support your sleep quality. There are other things that can indirectly support your sleep quality. I am going to share both. Direct is easier. First and foremost, you need to have a space without noise and as dark as possible. This is important because light and noise stimulate your brain and therefore distract and detract from sleep. You need to allow your brain to focus on the inside of your body, to do the best maintenance and repair work possible while you're sleeping. Anything that distracts your brain even a little bit, like a night-light or noise from a TV, will detract from your brain being at its best.

DO YOU HAVE DIFFICULTY SLEEPING?

You may have challenges sleeping, and whether you do or you don't, this next piece of advice is probably the most important one. You must have a routine sleep schedule. The closer you are to going to bed at the same time every day and waking up every morning, the better. Are you starting to pick up on *routine* as a general theme for all these simple habits?

Here is the easiest way to create your sleep routine. Have a consistent wake-up time. Science has made it very clear that seven to nine hours of sleep each night is the healthiest. Less than seven hours, on a regular basis, decreases your life expectancy. And more than nine hours on a regular basis, also decreases your life expectancy.

You can use an alarm clock to wake yourself up each morning at the same time. This is the primary target because if you start by only setting a bedtime, then you may not be tired, so you lay there awake and then you sleep in as a result. Then because you slept late, you are not tired again the next night. That's why setting your wake-up time is the primary target, the first thing to do. Then, you can reverse engineer it. Go backwards to determine what time you should go to bed at night based on your chosen ideal wake-up time. For example, let's assume you need to get up at 6:00 a.m. and let's aim for eight hours of sleep. That means you should have the lights out at 10:00 p.m. If you choose to get up at 7:00 a.m., target to have the lights out by 11:00 p.m. Simple!

Let's say that you fit in the category of "I'm not tired at night," or "I lay there, and my brain is running." I hear these scenarios often. Maybe you have aches and pains that make it difficult to sleep. Or maybe your brain just keeps running and you can't turn it off. Here is where the indirect sleep support techniques come in. You can't just magically make your pain go away when you're lying there. Unfortunately, your aches and pains are often amplified when you lay still because your brain isn't focused on other things, and so whatever is left (the aches and pains) gets more attention. This dynamic can make things even more difficult.

If you have aches and pains, they need to be addressed, and chiropractic care is your first stop. If you require more than just chiropractic care to resolve those aches and pains, then your chiropractor should be able to refer you to additional resources and health care options. In my experience, this need is rare because chiropractic care typically gives good results. Whatever avenue you choose, figure it out because chronic sleep deprivation will make things even worse. Medication is not a long-term solution, as it only decreases your symptoms at best. It does not solve the underlying issues. Drug-induced sleep is not healthy sleep. Seek solutions to the cause; don't settle on a legal drug habit to keep symptoms at bay.

If your mind is racing and you can't settle down, this can be tied to many causes. This is also more common than most people think. Again, you want to start with chiropractic care.

I have found, from helping thousands of patients over many years in our office, that when people have a certain subluxation in the top of their necks, it often correlates with sleep issues. Is it an adjustment for sleep? No, it's not. Remember that chiropractic just gets rid of what is wrong to leave you at your best. In this case, when you have a subluxation, particularly in the spine and particularly at the top of the neck (which is where your brain stem is sticking out of your skull), it is going to be a neurological irritant on your whole nervous system.

What does that mean? That means that at some level, your body will likely be in a state of fight or flight. Fight or flight is simply translated as a state of being when something has your body's attention, and there's an alarm that is going off that something is wrong. When that "alarm" is literally on your brain, or your brain stem in this example, which is part of the brain, then that's a pretty difficult alarm to ignore. In this case, it is an appropriate response. Your body is not doing anything wrong. It really is telling you there is something wrong.

This is why the first simple step is to visit a chiropractor to see if your sleep improves when your spine is aligned correctly. If spinal alignment turns out to be the answer, it will be the simplest and quickest solution to this issue.

Most issues have multiple contributing factors. I will get into your mindset or headspace in a later chapter. I will also get into exercise, since it also affects your sleep for better or worse. Remember what I have already talked about with food. We've discussed that certain food is healthy and nourishing and makes the body happy, and other food, if we want to call it that, is not so nourishing and not so healthy. This will also be an internal irritation to your body, which can result in making it difficult to get into a state of rest that healthy sleep requires.

CBD OIL

CBD oil is a safe and natural supplement that could possibly help you sleep. You need a good quality product for your safety and to determine its benefit for you. CBD naturally helps the body reduce inflammation. This is different from pharmaceuticals in that pharmaceuticals just mask the problem but actually do nothing for the cause of the inflammation. Drugs are like turning off the fire alarm but ignoring the fire. CBD is like water on a fire. We have carried high-quality CBD products at my office for years and it has been of great benefit to many patients. For more information on CBD, please visit www. ChrisPerron.com.

Overall, it is vital to make sure that you solve the sleep problem and it won't be through medication.

PILLOWS AND POSITIONS

People often ask about sleep positions as well as beds and pillows. They're great questions. And the answers are simple. Stomach sleeping is the one position that is terrible for you. It's the fact that you have to have your head turned sideways, and therefore your neck is twisted to one side or the other for hours on end, night after night. Typically, your arms will be up above the head, also jamming things up further in your neck and shoulders. And one leg is typically drawn up, making your hips and pelvis twisted as well. If you look like the chalk outline at a crime scene, that can't be good.

Sleeping flat on your back is ideal, for the exact opposite reasons. When you're on your back, everything is in place, everything is lined up, and your body is in an "anatomically neutral" position. No hands above your head though! Sleep in the same position as a corpse. Rest in peace!

If you find this difficult to do, here's a simple little tip. Take a full-size pillow and put it underneath your knees while you're lying on your back. This will prop your knees up, so they'll have a slight bend. Rest your legs completely on the pillow. By having a slight bend in your knees, it will accomplish two things. First, it takes a little pressure off your lower back muscles. For some, at least initially, you may feel tightness in your lower back when you lay flat on your back because it forces your hip flexors to extend. If you are like most, your hip flexors are too tight from sitting too much, and therefore it hurts to lay flat. The pillow under your knees is a good way to help your body to transition to sleeping on your back.

When you sleep on your back, you want to use one pillow under your head. Why? You don't want your head to be shoved up into the air. You want it in line with the rest of your body. Use one pillow simply for cushioning and not for support. A thinner pillow is best. If you feel like your head is being jutted forward, then that's a sign that you may have a pillow that's too thick.

Sleeping on your side is okay, depending on your issues, or lack thereof. Sleeping on your side can be okay or it could be irritating, but typically it's okay. You will want to switch sides periodically so that you aren't consistently pushing one shoulder or jamming one shoulder versus spending some time on each shoulder. This spreads the pressure, and that decreases the odds of creating problems. If you sleep on your side, the goal is to literally be on your side. You do not want your arms to be up above your head. You don't want to be laying with your head on your upper arm; although, on your hand is fine. Picture hugging your pillow or a teddy bear, that's where you want your arms to be. Pillow-wise, you'll need a thick enough pillow to fill in the width of your shoulder. You're looking for your head and neck to be perpendicular to your shoulders across your collarbones.

If you have a spouse or anybody else living in your house with you, lay on the pillow and have them look at you. Ask them to tell you if you're pretty close to your head and neck being perpendicular to your shoulders across your collarbones. It's difficult for you to be able to tell this by feel because your body may be trained and accustomed to being crooked. When you're actually in the correct position, initially that can feel crooked to you. Having an outside pair of eyes confirm what amount of pillow you need can be helpful. A large mirror could also work in a pinch.

Broad shoulders often need two pillows or at least a much thicker pillow. Shoulders that are not as broad may only need one pillow. Pillows come in lots of shapes and sizes, with a little effort you'll figure out the setup that works for you.

As a bonus, if you would like (this is not always necessary), you could choose to put a pillow between your knees as well. Your hips are wider than your knees; therefore, there's a natural gap between your knees. When you lay on your side, the top leg is naturally going to collapse down. If you find that it is pulling you forward and giving you a bit of a twist, then it is a good idea to stick a pillow between your knees. That will help you to avoid that twisted position and stay more in line.

The less strain you put on your body—the better or the fewer distractions your body has to tolerate as it's trying to do its nightly maintenance—the better you will be in the morning.

MATTRESSES

Mattresses are a regular source of blame at my office. My suggestion is to address all of the above first, including chiropractic care. It is magical that most of the time it is not the mattress when you address your part of the relationship.

As a general rule, most typical mattresses have a lifespan of eight to ten years. Good to keep in mind when determining when your mattress might be a contributing cause of your problems.

As far as mattress recommendations, I recommend Sleep Number. Especially if you have no idea what kind of mattress works best for you with regard to firmness as well as if you share a bed with someone else who may have different needs. The Sleep Number allows for experimentation over time to discover your "number," which correlates to firmness. I had one for many years and enjoyed it. However, once you know your "number," knowledge is power.

I switched to a latex mattress several years ago for its non-toxic qualities and was able to choose my ideal firmness because of the knowledge I gained from the Sleep Number. I love my bed for the comfort and enjoy knowing that I am not inhaling invisible toxic fumes every night as a bonus.

ACTION STEPS:

☐ Determine your ideal wake-up time, and from there, your ideal bedtime.

☐ Establish a nightly routine to be off all electronics at least thirty minutes before bedtime and do something relaxing like reading or drinking chamomile tea.

☐ Get rid of all lights and noises in your sleep environment.

☐ Choose a sleep position(s).

☐ Make sure you have a pillow game plan for your chosen position(s).

☐ After a couple of weeks, if you have problems, make sure you are addressing the other habits for indirect issues.

☐ Explore CBD options if needed at www.ChrisPerron.com.

☐ Explore mattress options if needed, and find additional resources at www.ChrisPerron.com.

RECAP: WHY SLEEP IS ESSENTIAL

Sleep is one of the most vital ingredients to being healthy. Begin with the plan outlined in this chapter to establish a routine. Simultaneously implement the other habits as they address many of the most common causes of sleep issues.

The Simple Plan is a package deal and the quality of your sleep is often an indicator of your overall health.

EXERCISE (BE ACTIVE!)

"You have to exercise, or at some point you will just break down."

—PRESIDENT BARACK OBAMA

TIPS FROM THE HULK

"Hey Lou!," my college roommate yelled across the gym as we walked in. It was my freshman year at the University of Miami and one of my roommates, Steve, was a local kid. He invited me to go work out at his gym off campus. Although I played a lot of sports, lifting weights was foreign to me. Next thing I knew, Steve was introducing me to the largest human being I had ever seen in person. His muscles had muscles and yet he looked really familiar. Then a lightbulb went off in my head and I realized it was *The Incredible Hulk*! It must have been the lack of green body paint that caused me to take a second to connect the dots. Of course, I played it cool and said hello but inside, I was like "Holy $%&^!" We all chatted for just a few moments. He had a great smile and gentle giant vibe to him that left me with a good impression.

Off we all went to work out. This gym was clean but it was like "Mama's House of Iron." No frills, just equipment and people who looked like they knew what they were doing. Since I was on the University of Miami Crew Team, I soon found myself gravitating toward the weighted row machine. I had not used this before, although it didn't seem complicated. I picked a weight, stuck the pin in the stack, grabbed the handle, and sat back to do my thing. A couple of reps in I suddenly felt a mammoth paw on my left shoulder and another in the middle of my back. You guessed it; it was The Hulk! Lou Ferrigno gently pulled my shoulders back while simultaneously pressing in on the middle of my back to straighten me up like I was in the uniform inspection line for Army ROTC.

"You need to keep your back just like this the whole time. Only your arms move. Go ahead and do a few reps." I did as I was told, of course, and it felt completely different. It felt like the best posture I could create. It also felt stronger, stable, and controlled with a more solid base that he helped me discover. "Hey, thanks, Lou! That feels really different. Better."

Lou responded, "The secret to working out is form. Don't worry about how much weight you use. That happens naturally. If your form is wrong, you'll hurt yourself and then you can't work out and you get nowhere. Keep it simple, work out the right way, and just keep showing up and putting in the effort."

He showed me a few more things, I thanked him, and we went our separate ways. That was the only time I saw Lou Ferrigno in person but I will keep his wisdom and generosity to share it for my lifetime.

JUST GET MOVING

Exercise carries a bad connotation with a lot of people, kind of like vegetables. We all know it is good for us and we should *but...*

Why don't we just call it being active, moving, or movement?

We all need to be physically active. The old saying, "Use it or lose it," is quite appropriate. In this chapter, I will outline a foundation of healthy activity so that you can have clarity on what would equate to enough activity, as well as which activities are best.

It doesn't have to be anything formal or exciting, unless you want it to be. What you need to do is have a list of ways to move your body that meets your needs. You need to make the list short, sweet, and—most of all—targeted to you, so it meets your needs. If you want to go above and beyond that, more power to you. However, let's at least get your needs met. If, for some crazy reason, we can combine your needs with some stuff that you enjoy, that would be even better, right? Let's try to achieve both.

Moving your body is good—even essential—for your health. Purposeful exercises train your body to move the way you would like it to move. I want you to really think about that. Keep in mind that it's not a matter of how heavy of a weight you can pick up. It's not even a matter of even how fast we can go, unless you're training for the Olympics. I'm not. It's about creating patterns of motion in your muscles that are appropriate. You have likely heard the term "muscle memory," but this is not actually a thing. What really happens is your brain creates memories of patterns it gives to your muscles in the form of instructions. The more often you move a certain way, the brain also reinforces this pattern and becomes more efficient at it. This is the goal of all athletes when training for a sport: to perform a certain set of actions at a high level. There is one small issue we all run into, and it is training our brain to instruct our muscles to perform a compensating pattern, also known as the wrong pattern. You see, our muscles don't think; they just do their best. So when you are slouching, know that you are training your brain to instruct your muscles to perform that pattern.

Changing the muscle patterns is the part that takes the most time and effort when working with patients through chiropractic. I can adjust and realign your joints. In relative terms, that is the easy part. It is getting your body to get used to having your joints lined up *correctly,* which takes time. This requires old compensating patterns to shift to patterns of working the correct way again. This takes not only time but consistency in performing the correct motions the right way. The better the muscles are supporting the proper alignment, the more stable the joint will be.

When we move, chemical reactions take place. Think of a metal hinge on a gate door that has not been opened in years. What happens when you try to open that gate? Initially it will be stiff and it might take quite a bit of effort to get it to move at all. There's a reason for this. It's the same reason your body needs to move. Your muscles and joints are made for one purpose, to move. If you don't move your joints, they, too, will "rust." Movement keeps you healthy. Movement tells your brain, "Hey! We need some lubrication for those knee joints. Hey! We could use a little bit more oxygen down here. And hey, we can use more blood flow down over there, and some nutrients to replenish me and keep things ready to move."

That's what good health is. If you don't stimulate your body in a way that tells your brain to give you some good stuff, then your brain starts just focusing on what we *do* tell it.

"Just exist, no need for maintenance. I never use my hip anyway." For the best results, you want to purposefully tell your brain what you want. I'm going to give you the basics, because that's how I like to keep it. If you want to build upon the foundation I will share, then great. But making sure you have a solid foundation is your first step. I strongly advise that you at least do what I'm about to describe.

BE THE TORTOISE, NOT THE HARE

Your goal is to do some form of exercise/activity every single day. Consistency outweighs intensity; slow and steady wins the race. It's true. Every day, exercise for thirty minutes as your norm, or twenty minutes minimum in a pinch.

You'll need a couple of different options. Primarily, you need some form of cardiovascular exercise, something that will get your heart rate up, and maybe even get a little sweat going. There are many ways to accomplish this. You can include a brisk walk, ride a bike, use various exercise machines if you go to a gym, take water aerobics, or swim. As you can see, there are many ways to get the job done.

Ideally, choose at least two activities for the best results. Find a couple that you prefer more than others so that you don't become a "one-trick pony." It is not ideal to do the same exercise repeatedly, again and again and again and again. Why? Your body and your brain are smart. They get used to doing the same motion, and they learn how to do it better, and better, and more efficiently. What does that translate to? Over time, you actually get less of a workout by doing the same activity because your body just learns how to do it better and more efficiently. Now, it's a good thing that your body learns how to do those physical activities better. That's part of the point of doing the activities. However, in the long run, your body needs variety to keep your brain guessing and paying attention for the best long-term results.

Choose two different activities that you know you could do consistently starting tomorrow, ideally one outdoors and one indoors so that you are covered regardless of weather.

On days when the weather isn't to your liking, it is good to have an indoor option. Getting outside and breathing fresh air is something we can all use more of so having at least one outside option is important as well. It can be as simple as taking a walk. Whatever way works for you is fine. Just aim for thirty minutes every day.

By the way, did you know that more is not always better? There's no point in killing yourself unless you are training for a specific activity, like a race. Thirty minutes is plenty when you do it consistently. But if it's a nice day and you want to go for a longer stroll, enjoy it!

Along with the cardiovascular exercise that makes your

lungs and heart happy and healthy, you'll also need some resistance training. This comes in many different forms as well: classic weights, resistance bands, or best of all, your own body weight.

You need something that makes you strain your muscles a little bit. There are a couple of resistance exercises that I believe everyone should do, and what I have found is that most people don't do them unless I share them.

FORM IS KEY!

Remember what Lou taught me: form is key! The two most important movements are "rows" and "lat pull-downs." I provide video demonstrations of how to do these on my website www.ChrisPerron.com. If you go to the gym already, just ask a trainer to show you how to do these two moves. Rows and lat pull-downs both end with pulling your shoulders back and down, which reinforces good posture. We can all use that, especially in modern lifestyles with computer use, driving, and everything else that pulls us forward.

Push-ups and planks are fantastic for your body as well. You want to concentrate on form over quantity and speed. In other words, focus primarily on form. For push-ups and planks, do two sets of your maximum ability. Meaning when your form starts to go then you know that set is done.

How simple is this? If you were to do these moves (rows, lat pull-downs, push-ups, and planks) consistently, three times each week plus the cardiovascular exercise, in my opinion, you're done. That should reinforce a solid foundation for your health. It's all you'd need to do!

Please ask your chiropractor which exercises are best for you to train your muscles out of compensating patterns. If you want to do more or different exercises, I recommend asking your chiropractor as well. Depending on your history and your level of stability in certain areas of your body, some exercises can be hazardous, and your chiropractor should be able to speak to that.

In review, the simple step of moving and using your body is first and foremost about frequency. It's not about intensity. That is why it is a habit. Choose to create this habit, put your body in motion each day, and go from there.

SKYDIVING WITH PRESIDENT GEORGE H. W. BUSH!

George H. W. Bush is an example of someone who stayed healthy by moving well into their later years. George, who was Vice President of the United States and later became President, has a connection with me. My family and I got to meet him when he was Vice President. Here is the picture; I, of course, am the dashing young man up front.

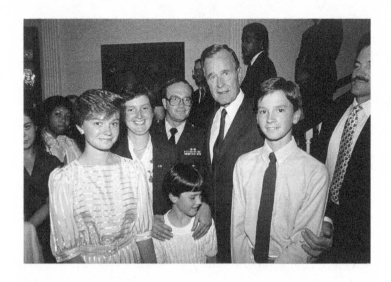

We were celebrating his birthday with him at the US Embassy in Ottawa, Canada. Can you believe my dad got stationed in Canada for three years and I got to meet Queen Elizabeth II *and* Vice President Bush?! What are the odds of that?

I remember two things about him. He was quite friendly and had a big hand when I shook it. What I have always found intriguing about him is that he had a tradition of going sky-diving on his birthday. He did this into his nineties!

Just like Queen Elizabeth II and her nutritional habits, George H. W. Bush was physically active into his nineties. Both are examples of great longevity. They didn't both just exist for a long time; they lived life fully and Queen Elizabeth II is still going strong.

THE PLAN IN ACTION

My father implemented this step during those three days I was visiting their house after my mother's heart attack. His choice was riding his bike. The weather was good, so he hopped on his bike, and I hopped on my mom's bike, and we went for a cruise around his neighborhood. The first day we went about three miles. I will let you know that he hadn't exercised in quite a while, but he did fine! He continued to ride three miles per day.

My dad, an Army veteran, can be very disciplined when he's got a plan. That pretty much describes most of us on some level, and that's the point of having a plan and why I am sharing it with you as I did with my own parents. You likely do better with a clear plan, too.

I don't think my dad has missed a day yet, and it's been over two years since he started. Now, he rides over six miles per day. Going to the gym has been a challenge due to the COVID-19 pandemic, so he and my mother do their resistance training at home with resistance bands, as well as planks and push-ups. My mother wanted me to check her form on a recent visit to my house, so she got on the floor and started her plank. Her form was quite good. Then something surprising happened: she just kept holding her plank. She held her plank in good form for well over a minute on her forearms and toes. The real deal plank. Not bad for a year removed from having a "widowmaker" heart attack and being seventy years young!

If you have any physical issues as you begin this process, before you start, or after you start, then definitely check in with your chiropractor. We are trained for this, and we can advise you on what to do and what not to do, and sometimes just what not to do temporarily. Your plan will evolve over time as you improve your health and fitness levels. If you have any aches and pains, they could prevent you from doing certain exercises, or even be harmful. Don't cover up your symptoms with a pill; let your chiropractor help you find a real solution.

Don't let excuses linger for not exercising. You may have a valid excuse, but you need a plan to figure out what you can do, not just what you can't do. If you aren't sure what to do, then seek help from a trained professional, another brain who can creatively and safely help you to figure out how to find a starting point. Figuring out that first plan can be the hardest, but after that it is just tweaks and changes. Action always outweighs everything else. Your body will give you feedback; just listen to it and proceed accordingly. If you don't do anything, you won't get the feedback. If you don't get feedback, then you don't know what's working, good or bad. This feedback is crucial in navigating your choice of activities and creating a nice, steady rhythm that is best for you.

MARTHA STEWART

For anyone who thinks you are too old to exercise, please don't buy into that. Let me share a quick story that I think was kind of cool. I was attending an event at Carnegie Hall in New York City and met Martha Stewart. I think we all know who Martha Stewart is, and at this stage of her life she's not exactly a spring chicken. In fact, she's in her early eighties. And yet she's full of energy, she's on new TV shows all the time, with different angles, and by all accounts she is healthy and energetic.

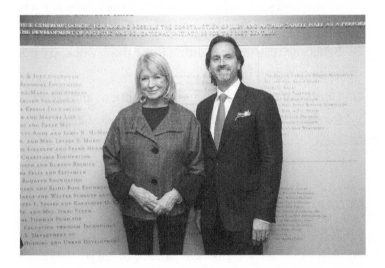

I asked Martha, "What do you do to take care of yourself?"

She told me that fitness is intertwined in her daily routine. She shared that she has a large property in Connecticut, where she lives, and she walks the perimeter of her property each morning. She also enjoys gardening. That's nothing over the top. It's pretty simple. Martha said that by doing these things she gets to connect with nature, get some fresh air, and it just sets her mind for the day.

ACTION STEPS:

☐ Determine your two cardiovascular exercise options and work towards thirty minutes/day.

☐ Determine where you can do your rows and lat pull-downs and seek instruction through my videos at www. ChrisPerron.com and/or from a trainer.

☐ Schedule resistance training three days/week; try not to do two days in a row.

☐ Check out your push-up and plank options and the form for each through my video training at www.ChrisPerron. com.

RECAP: WHY WE NEED TO BE ACTIVE

Consider the simplicity of taking a walk like Martha Stewart. It doesn't take a lot, as I said, and I can tell you firsthand that she is an excellent example of great health and longevity. Add a few minutes of resistance training as well and you will be doing great.

You can do it, too. Get started today!

SELF-LOVE (CULTIVATE THE MINDSET TO SUCCEED)

"Our deepest fear is not that we are inadequate. Our deepest fear is that we are powerful beyond measure. It is our light, not our darkness that most frightens us. We ask ourselves, 'Who am I to be brilliant, gorgeous, talented, fabulous?' Actually, who are you not to be? You are a child of God. Your playing small does not serve the world. There is nothing enlightened about shrinking so that other people won't feel insecure around you. We are all meant to shine, as children do. We were born to manifest the glory of God that is within us. It's not just in some of us; it's in everyone. And as we let our light shine, we unconsciously give other people permission to do the same. As we are liberated from our own fear, our presence automatically liberates others."

—MARIANNE WILLIAMSON, "OUR DEEPEST FEAR"

OVERCOMING OBSTACLES

It was the summer of 1989. I was sixteen years old and was applying to go to the United States Naval Academy in Annapolis, Maryland. I wanted to become a Navy SEAL. My father's career was in the Army, so logically I wanted to join the Navy. My thinking was if I was going into the military, I wanted to be the best-trained, most badass soldier I could be. It was a matter of self-preservation as well as "being all I could be." Oops, that's the Army's slogan.

I was in a gymnasium at Fort Belvoir, just outside of Washington, DC, on a summer day. My friend Steve and I had driven there to participate in the physical aptitude test with other academy candidates. I was athletic and did well. I remember that a general walked into the gym right as it was my turn to do pull-ups. He was in full uniform with ribbons and medals galore. I stepped up and cranked out over double the pull-ups I had ever done. Eleven.

A couple of weeks later, I was at the hospital at Fort Belvoir going through the last step in the process, a medical exam. This of course was a formality. I could not have been healthier and went through their tests with great ease and confidence. The last part of the exam was a color vision test. I thought to myself, "This should be fun. I've never done one of these before." I sat down in the room with the doctor, and he pulled out a spiral-bound book that had fourteen pages and they were thick, hard pages like each one was a book cover. He opened it up and there was a circle of dots. He asked, "What do you see?" I looked and responded, "A circle of dots." He asked, "What else?" I said, "Nothing." Then, he flipped the page. Same question, same answer. By the time he got to the fourth page, I laughingly responded, "You're kidding, right? There is nothing else there." He continued through the fourteen pages and closed the book. He turned to me and said, "Son, I am sorry to tell you that your dream of going to the Naval Academy just ended." I was color blind.

Apparently, they want you to be able to see the dots on the radar and stuff. I still look back and am surprised at how well I took this news. The reality is that I would want to see everything on a radar as well. Let alone anything else that may be beneficial to not getting myself or the people around me killed.

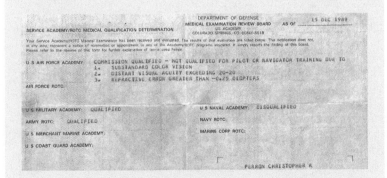

Clearly, I was facing a significant moment in my life where I needed a mindset to overcome this setback and succeed.

DEVELOPING THE RIGHT MINDSET

Mindset is a deeply personal subject with endless avenues to explore. I believe the point is to explore as many as possible. It has been said that the greatest knowledge is to know oneself. I have spent the last fifteen years diving into trying to figure out how and why I "tick."

Some people, who typically have not embarked on such a quest, might view this as self-absorbed. But if you do, let me tell you that it is the exact opposite. If you try to figure yourself out, you will understand how you interact with others better. You will learn the good and the bad. Then, and only then, do you have a chance to make a conscious choice to improve your approach to better your relationships. It will always start with your relationship with yourself. That is often the least comfortable relationship to explore. But it is the only one you really can control, so it is well worth the effort.

I like the phrase "self-love." You need to feel you are worth the effort of the other six habits to likely implement them, let alone sustain them for your benefit. A phrase a mentor of mine once shared is, "You can never out-love another person's love for themselves." Really take that in. You can't override someone else's challenges no matter how hard you try. *They* must do it. More so, flip it around and put yourself in the role of the recipient of love in that quote. You can't accept love from anyone else more than you accept your own love of yourself. That is mind-blowing to me and I have also found it to be true.

Love is an action to me. It is what we do, not just a feeling. The Simple Plan is an act of self-love. In essence, this is a practical guide as to how to express love for yourself. Now if you are healthier, and almost by default happier, then what are you bringing to the people around you? That's right; you are bringing love.

You will run into challenges in life. That is human. There is another quote from Tony Robbins that can put a spin on self-pity and a victim mentality: "Life is always happening for you, not to you."

Life is a series of circumstances. Some good, some bad. In the end, it just is. You can't control your environment. The only thing you have influence over is yourself. Let's focus on the things you *can* control, not on the things you can't.

HOW CAN YOU APPROACH GROWTH?

There are endless books already written on the topic of personal growth and I recommend you dive in and see what you discover. Audiobooks in the car are great and reading a motivating book versus watching the news is also a great way to feed your mind.

I do want to share a few things you can begin to incorporate today that are proven to calm the mind. A calm mind is a well-functioning mind.

MEDITATION

I meditate every day and I recommend that you do the same. There are many approaches to meditation, but I like to keep it simple. This is supposed to clear the mind, not give you something else to focus on.

The simplest and most effective approach I have found is a simple, breath-focused approach. You need to sit. Either on the floor with your legs crossed or in a chair with both feet flat on the floor. Then lay your hands palm up on your thighs at a comfortable distance, somewhere around your knees. Sit up perfectly straight with perfect posture as this puts your body at ease and allows you to breathe freely. Now close your eyes and start inhaling slowly into your nose and exhaling out of your mouth. Focus on the air going in and going out. Thoughts will soon come into your consciousness, what you have to do that day, what happened yesterday, did I put the laundry in the dryer...? Let the thoughts be there, since you can't stop them anyway. But gently bring your focus back to the breathing. Do this for ten minutes every day.

The process of this meditation allows your brain to touch

on all those thoughts. It gives your mind the feeling that you have given it attention so you can now relax about it. Ideally, you should try to meditate until there are no more thoughts that show up. Like you checked all the boxes. If done consistently, it will help calm your mind.

MINIMIZE MEDIA (SOCIAL AND MAINSTREAM)

Try to keep this to a minimum. There is rarely anything positive and every thought we take in adds up. If you are watching the news all day or the latest scandal, then you can expect to be more stressed out, even though you have no direct control over 99 percent of it. Would you not benefit society better by being a source of positivity instead of getting caught up in the negativity? The reality is that fear sells. It is a fact so that is why most media is negative, which is fear based. Whether it is selling you a product or just getting you to tune in more so the source gets more ad buys, someone is benefitting from your attention. Ask yourself if you and the people you encounter each day are benefiting as well.

WORK TOWARD YOUR GOALS

As I was helping my parents to implement this step, I suggested they choose a goal that would build them as people. I suggested that they needed to be working toward something. They have travel goals of places they want to visit as well as experiences to have with their kids and grandkids. Here is a tip: if you don't necessarily meet the goal on the level that you wanted to, that's okay! The idea is to be working *toward* something, and you are still going to be better off for having grown in that direction. As the saying goes, "If you aim for the moon and miss, you may hit a star."

As you write out your goals (yes, actually write them down to reinforce the thought), write them in a positive way. For instance, my mother could have an understandable goal of not having another heart attack. I support that, too. However, it would be better to flip it to a goal of being healthy and active enough to take her grandchildren to Disney World. See what I mean? One is positive and the other is avoidance and based in fear. Same result, different perspective. If you remind yourself of what you are afraid of regularly, it will actually reinforce the fear. Choose to reinforce the positive!

PURPOSE AND PLANNING

There also needs to be a purpose to your days. It does not have to be a profound purpose, but a productive one. We all feel more at peace when we have a sense of being in control of our lives. Total control is not possible, but you have a lot of influence. Create a Three Accomplishments a Day Checklist. Every evening write down three things that you want to accomplish the next day. It could be things like work out, cook dinner, get the oil changed, or call your mom. It does not have to be profound. Cut yourself some slack. Try to choose things you know you need to do but may have been putting off or that you know are good for you, but you don't love it, so you seem to come up with excuses quite often.

Establish the routine of reviewing your list each evening. Physically cross off the things you did and then write down your three for the next day. You will feel a sense of accomplishment. You may be productive already, but by physically taking a moment to do this routine, you will impact yourself psychologically and it will fuel your passion for the next day.

It's that simple.

ACTION STEPS:

☐ Meditate daily.

☐ Start the Three Accomplishments a Day Checklist routine.

☐ Take time for yourself; think and write out what is important to you in life, and then start crafting your life steadily to include more and more of it.

☐ Begin the habit of reading or listening to books on personal growth. There is an entire section at Barnes & Noble devoted to it. I didn't know either.

☐ Journal daily—Write about anything or make it a gratitude journal and write three things you are grateful for each day.

RECAP: WHY DO YOU NEED TO LOVE YOURSELF?

I had the privilege of going to an event in New York City, where I got to meet and talk with Ice-T, the actor and musician, and his wife, Coco. Both are big personalities but refreshingly down-to-earth and friendly people. We were talking about goals and hard work when Ice-T shared this very simple quote: "Remember that nobody else wakes up with your dream."

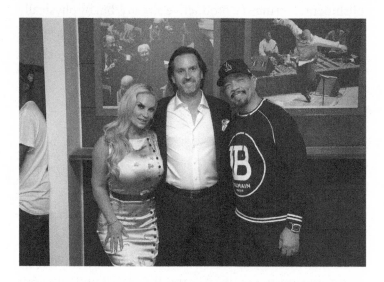

Whatever your dreams are, the one person who must make it happen is you. The clearer you are about your dreams, the more support you're going to find for achieving it. If you don't have a dream, or if you don't have a clear idea of what you want, where you want to be, and how you want it to be, then you are just along for the ride and you get what you get. Like a ship without a rudder. By identifying what is important to you in life, you will unlock the most powerful motivator to achieving your dreams.

HYDRATION (DRINK UP!)

"I believe water is the only drink for a wise man."

—HENRY DAVID THOREAU

Kylie Jenner and Jennifer Aniston swear by water as a staple to their health and beauty regime. Hydrating your skin from the inside out is what Kylie says. Tom Brady drinks up to double what I recommend below (unless you, too, are a professional athlete, my suggestions should be sufficient). These successful people rely on their body and their minds to create the success that they have had over an extended period of time. Water is one of the secret ingredients to looking, feeling, and functioning at your best.

Drinking water seems so easy, but yet many people don't take in enough water for proper hydration. And I do mean literally water, good old H_2O. Just because something is a liquid does not mean it hydrates your body or supports your health.

HOW MUCH WATER DO YOU NEED PER DAY?

This is pretty simple, and it's an answer that is personalized for you. Take your body weight in pounds, and then divide that number in half. That's how many ounces of water you should be drinking—every day. For example, if you weigh 128 pounds, 128 divided in half is 64. You would need 64 ounces, or half a gallon. If you are 200 pounds, divide it in half and you need 100 ounces of water per day. More would not be better and anything extreme is usually not a good thing, so just target your number.

From a practical standpoint, you need to be able to measure how much water you're drinking, in order to be consistent. I have found that it is difficult to track based on the number of glasses of water you drink each day, since some glasses are smaller than others. If you're drinking water based on the number of glasses a day, there's a little issue with how to keep track because all glasses are different. How can you keep count consistently? What size is your glass compared to my glass? There can be a lot of variables that come into play. The more variables, the higher the odds of not reaching this goal and just making your life harder.

SIMPLE STRATEGIES

Here are two simple strategies for ensuring you're drinking enough water.

THE PITCHER METHOD

If you are at home much of your day, even if you're in and out of the house but you're generally at home a lot, it's simple. Grab a pitcher or some sort of water container and use a form of measurement to figure out how much it holds. You could use a measuring cup, an empty water bottle, or anything that will help you figure out how many ounces the container holds.

When I taught this to my parents, they pulled out two similarly sized pitchers, each held sixty-four ounces. So with that, they each had a pitcher, his and hers. In the morning, they fill them up with water, but not tap water.

Please drink some form of filtered water. You want to get filtered water somehow. There are plenty of natural grocery stores that have a filtered water station where you can get one-gallon, three-gallon, or five-gallon jugs. I go to my local Whole Foods to get water and it costs a whopping thirty-nine cents a gallon. It can be quite cost friendly if you find a place like that. At the least, an at-home filter system like Brita would still be better than straight tap water.

My parents fill their pitchers up and then they both need to get through them by the end of the day. As I advised my mom and dad, you want to look at your pitcher periodically throughout the day. If you drink some water with your meals, and you have a few glasses of water throughout the day, you'll drink that pitcher. By midday, you'll want your pitcher to be at least half empty to try and keep a steady pace. In their particular case, they needed more than sixty-four ounces per day, based on their weight at that time. So the water they drank with meals was separate from the pitcher to increase the overall total. This does not need to be exact, just close and most importantly consistent.

Drinking water is like watering a lawn. Your body is similar. You don't want to just dump a gallon of water all at once. It won't do the lawn, or your body, as much good. You're not going to get as much soaking. If you dump a bucket of water on dry ground, what happens? Most of it runs off. That's why consistency is important. Slow and steady wins the race once again. By steadily putting water in your body during the day, that's how your body gains the most benefit from it.

THE BOTTLE METHOD

If you are like me, and you have a job outside the house, and you are going to be out for most of the day, there's another simple way to get the water you need: hit the bottle.

You need to use a water bottle. Preferably, use one that is like a sports bottle. That way it should hold twenty to thirty ounces. Figure out exactly how much it holds, and then do the quick math for how many bottles it takes to reach your goal. In our office, we give out high-quality water bottles as a thank you gift to all the kind people who are willing to share their stories as testimonials online. These bottles hold twenty-three ounces. If you need to drink sixty-four ounces of water, then that is three bottles per day. If you are like me, you need to drink four bottles each day.

It's simple. In the morning, fill it up. Drink it with meals, sip on it throughout the day, keep it with you. By midday, with lunch, you should be finished with half of your daily water goal. If not, then drink up and catch up. The water bottle gives you a visual reminder of where you are with your goal throughout the day, and that makes it simple to track and reach your daily goal. I also recommend a see-through bottle so that you have a visual of how much is in the bottle at any given time. This is an easy way to be reminded that you need to drink up or fill up.

There are a couple of valid concerns people have mentioned to me over the years. There are concerns about spending all day in the bathroom. Well, you might at first, and I do mean that. Let's go back to the analogy of dumping a bucket of water on dry ground. If you're drinking as much water as I described and you are in the bathroom often, that likely means you need to keep drinking all that water. Typically, it is because your body is not used to that amount and your insides are that dry ground, at first. But just like dry ground the water starts to sink in and saturate and as it does, it will allow for better absorption.

If frequent urination is a concern for you, then you should consult your doctor to determine the cause.

RINSE YOUR INNARDS

Another thing that water does is it rinses your body from the inside. Your kidneys are filters, and so is your liver and gallbladder. When you put something as pure as filtered water in your body, it's like rinsing the dirt off dirty dishes or dirty garden tools.

One basic sign of your hydration level is the color of your urine. It should be close to clear. Not cloudy and not dark yellow; that is not good. Your urine should be on the clearer side. If it's dark in color, or if it smells, those are warning signs that you do not drink enough water and possibly have kidney problems and your doctor should be aware of this. The color of your urine makes for a simple barometer that you can tell for yourself how things are going inside you.

It is simple chemistry. The more colored (darker) your urine is, the more stuff your body is excreting in a concentrated amount. A steady intake of water is what puts the least strain on your body by steadily rinsing out the garbage at a constant pace, which should not allow for buildup.

OTHER DRINKS

People frequently ask about drinking other beverages and liquids. I refer you to the chemical basis that water is H_2O, two hydrogen atoms and one oxygen atom attached together. Water is three simple little atoms, making one simple little molecule. One of the most basic things for our body to evaluate and process. Coffee is a dehydrator. Do you know that if you drink more than a cup or two each day, you will need to increase the amount of water you drink to offset the coffee?

The benefit of following the simple plan I suggest is this: how much of *anything* can you drink in a day? If you are purposely drinking half your body weight in ounces in water, then you don't leave much time for drinking other things.

If you want a glass of juice, it should be organic and not have high fructose corn syrup added to it, as many do. Organic juice is ideal. If you look at the label it should say "orange juice" and that is all. Short glasses are made for juice; big, tall glasses are made for water. I enjoy having a glass of wine, and I already mentioned I like to have a cup or two of coffee in the morning. I share this not to illustrate that if

I can get away with it then you can; but instead, my example demonstrates that this water plan is not the end of the world. It is a matter of quantity.

Also, do you know that alcohol is dehydrating? Like drinking coffee, a glass or two of alcohol will not put a dent in your water plan. When someone's hungover, it's because they dehydrated the heck out of their brain and that's what gives them a headache.

Soda is just horrible for your body. If you still drink soda, do yourself a favor and stop. That may be harder than you think since soda is made to be addictive. It's right up there with cigarettes. As far as I'm concerned, it is one of the worst things you can have, and diet soda is even worse than regular soda. Put it in the category of bad for you "food" that you consume once in a blue moon, if at all.

ACTION STEPS:

☐ Determine your target number by calculating half your body weight in ounces.
☐ Choose a strategy—pitcher or water bottle.
☐ Start to phase out or just quit drinking other liquids; make them the exception.

RECAP: WHY WATER IS SO IMPORTANT FOR HEALTH

You are a living being and your nervous system is a complex electrical system. You need water for survival. It is one of the easiest habits to implement, so get started today. A personal tip on substituting out alcohol and soda is to drink sparkling water. You get the bubbles for texture but that is it. I am a San Pelligrino fan and I can buy a case of twelve for the same price as a decent bottle of pinot noir. Drink up!

CONCLUSION

"If you focus on results, you will never change. If you focus on change, you will get results."

—JACK DAVIS

As I was getting close to publishing this book, I decided I needed to do my 90 Day Transformation Program in its entirety, the same as my parents did so that I could fully relate to what your experience will be like. I was not targeting weight loss since I was already down ten pounds in four months when I started to be more consistent with these habits and went from my past decade average of 196 to 186 pounds. I am 6'0" tall, so that is a reasonable weight for my size, but I knew I would be healthier for having followed The Simple Plan completely and that is always a worthwhile reason.

Over the course of the three months, my patients were asking me what I was doing because I was shedding the belly padding I still had left rather rapidly. There were comments on my mood, even though I have always been a pretty lighthearted, friendly person. Comments included, "How are you getting younger?" and "Can I have what you're having?" A few patients even expressed concern, wondering if I was okay. My answer to all was that I simply started following my own advice better. I am forty-nine years old and I am as fit as when I graduated from chiropractic school at twenty-three. I bottomed out at 172 pounds towards the end of the ninety days. That means I ran out of fat to shed. I have increased my food intake even more to keep up with my renewed exercise level. The most interesting thing that I experienced is that I like being this way! I have increased energy, look better, feel better, and it was all from doing no more than what is described in this book. With one exception. I work out pretty hard. P90X is my routine of choice. But that only gives me muscle tone, not all the other health benefits including shedding the extra fat. There is a saying in the bodybuilding world, "You get strong in the gym but lean in the kitchen." You do not need to do P90X; my mother was doing rehab from her heart attack. Her weight loss and improved health was driven by the other habits. Now I am a walking, talking testimonial myself and people are surprised by my unintended before and after pictures. The before shot (196 pounds) was a summer ago but reflects my entire forties. The after shot (172 pounds) was just a picture at the beach a couple weeks after following the 90 Day Transformation Program. They were not intended to be "before and after shots."

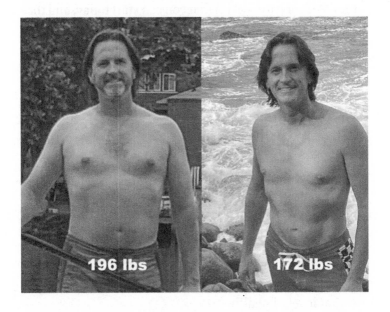

196 lbs   172 lbs

This is a Simple Plan with extreme results.

There you have it. All 7 Habits for Healthy Living.

I believe you can implement any of these habits if you really choose to.

Remember that it is a journey. Judge yourself on progress, not just the end result. These habits are not going to be easy to do at first, depending on where you are starting from, but with effort I believe you can do it.

I recognize a plan, even a great plan, is useless if not implemented. Therefore, here's a recap of the 7 Habits for Healthy Living. Remember, you don't have to do these in order. Pick one (or more!) that you can start today, and then build on your momentum. Give yourself a clean slate with the first two, and then reinforce it with the FRESH five!

ACTION STEPS:

SIMPLE HABIT 1: INCORPORATE CHIROPRACTIC CARE

☐ Write down your definition of success as you see things right now. Don't worry about what you think is realistic or not, make your wish list.

☐ Example: I would like to be pain free, fully functional, and have some knowledge on what I can do to sustain that level of health.

☐ Have this conversation with your chiropractor to make sure you are both on the same page. We are not mind readers. This can help us to help you.

☐ If you currently don't have a chiropractor, get one. Use the tips above to get started. You must include this foundational habit of The Simple Plan.

SIMPLE HABIT 2: RESTORE YOUR GUT AND BRAIN

☐ Start using only organic extra virgin olive oil (OEVOO) in your home.

☐ Take a high-quality omega-3 supplement daily. Nordic Naturals DHA 1000 is what I prescribe to my patients. (Adults) 2/day for sustaining health, 4/day if trying to improve your health. *As always, check with your doctor

☐ Enroll in the Gut and Brain Restoration Program—www. ChrisPerron.com.

SIMPLE HABIT 3: FOOD (FEED YOUR BODY)

☐ Go through your kitchen and get rid of everything that does not fit what I described.

☐ For the 90 Day Transformation Program, that means no bread, pasta, alcohol, soda, or anything else processed (made for you).

☐ Have a smoothie for lunch, snack in the afternoon, and dinner. Vega ONE's best pricing is typically online.

☐ Make your menu.

☐ Go grocery shopping for the ingredients for several of the meals on your menu.

☐ Begin intermittent eating. Choose your eight hour eating window and begin.

☐ Decide if you know how to make twelve meals and look into cooking lessons, helpful tips, and further support at www.ChrisPerron.com.

SIMPLE HABIT 4: REST (PRIORITIZE REST AND RECOVERY)

☐ Determine your ideal wake-up time, and from there, your ideal bedtime.

☐ Establish a nightly routine to be off all electronics at least thirty minutes before bedtime and do something relaxing like reading or drinking chamomile tea.

☐ Get rid of all lights and noises in your sleep environment.

☐ Choose a sleep position(s).

☐ Make sure you have a pillow game plan for your chosen position(s).

☐ After a couple of weeks, if you have problems, make sure you are addressing the other habits for indirect issues.

☐ Explore CBD options if needed at www.ChrisPerron. com.

☐ Explore mattress options if needed, and find additional resources at www.ChrisPerron.com.

SIMPLE HABIT 5: EXERCISE (BE ACTIVE!)

☐ Determine your two cardiovascular exercise options and work towards thirty minutes/day.

☐ Determine where you can do your rows and lat pull-downs and seek instruction through my videos at www. ChrisPerron.com and/or from a trainer.

- ☐ Schedule for resistance training three days/week; try not to do two days in a row.
- ☐ Check out your push-up and plank options and the form for each through my video training at www.ChrisPerron.com.

SIMPLE HABIT 6: SELF-LOVE (CULTIVATE THE MINDSET TO SUCCEED)

- ☐ Meditate daily.
- ☐ Start the Three Accomplishments a Day Checklist routine.
- ☐ Take time for yourself; think and write out what is important to you in life, and then start crafting your life steadily to include more and more of it.
- ☐ Begin the habit of reading or listening to books on personal growth. There is an entire section at Barnes & Noble devoted to it. I didn't know either.
- ☐ Journal daily—Write about anything or make it a gratitude journal and write three things you are grateful for each day.

SIMPLE HABIT 7: HYDRATION (DRINK UP!)

- ☐ Determine your target number by calculating half your body weight in ounces.
- ☐ Choose a strategy—pitcher or water bottle.

☐ Start to phase out or just quit drinking other liquids; make them the exception.

Starting is half the journey, so choose a couple of the habits that will be the easiest for you and begin from there. Just move forward, and as you notice small changes I believe you will become motivated to add more and stay on the path of progress. Your results will be relative to your effort. For big results, you will need to follow the entire plan and do the 90 Day Transformation Program.

YOU'RE INVITED!

I would like to invite you to continue this conversation online at www.ChrisPerron.com.

Additional resources can be found there to support you in your journey. I will add content regularly to grow this resource to serve you. Food and self-love, in particular, are endless subjects to explore but all the other habits will be discussed in greater depth as I continue to receive feedback from people like you. Please send questions to me directly at Dr@ChrisPerron.com.

The Simple Plan has worked *every* time to improve health. It is not the latest fad; it is tried and true, but with guidance to leverage the benefits for yourself through implementation. Be confident that it will benefit you and get moving toward your best self!

Here's to your health!

ACKNOWLEDGMENTS

I have been so fortunate to have MANY people in my life contribute to my benefit.

For all of you, I am sincerely grateful!

This is the short list.

My parents for their ever-present support while giving me the space to grow.

The US Army for transferring my father (and us) every two to three years, which provided me the opportunity to appreciate people being different, yet the same.

Drs. Andy Smith, Paul Curcio, and Tammy Cashion for hiring my mother as your office manager and introducing me to Chiropractic at just the right time.

Dr. Arlan Fuhr, for inventing and developing the Activator Methods Chiropractic Technique and then allowing me to be an instructor for over twenty years and hone my skills.

Drs. Wayne Comeau, Thomas DeVita, Chris Colloca, Steven Levy, Michael DeRose, and Phillip Pavkov for being instrumental in connecting me to Activator Methods.

Drs. Frank Sovinsky, Douglas Sea, and Cecile Thackeray and everyone of my DC Mentors comrades for introducing me to a path of personal and professional growth.

Drs. Tom Wetzen, Will Sonak, Michelle Rose, Ray Tuck, and Jay Greenstein as well as Julie Connolly and ALL of my Unified Virginia Chiropractic Association colleagues.

Clint Arthur, mentor/coach, for guiding me to make this book happen!